The Psoas Book
By Liz Koch

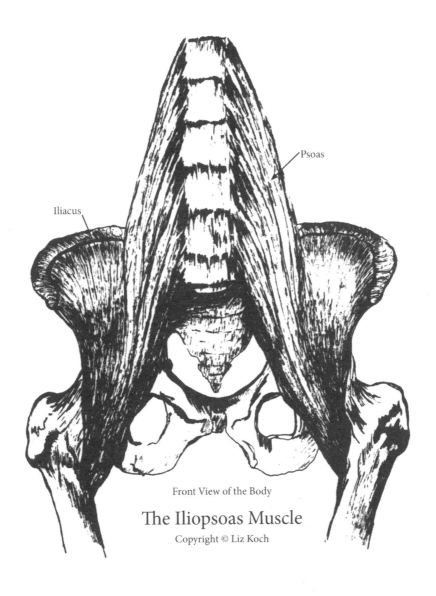

Psoas

Iliacus

Front View of the Body

The Iliopsoas Muscle

Copyright © Liz Koch

The Psoas Book
30th Anniversary Revised Edition

For wholesale information and/or requests please contact:
Guinea Pig Publications
P.O. Box 1226
Felton, CA 95018
(831)-335-1851
info@guineapigpub.com
For retail orders and workshop information please visit
www.coreawareness.com

Library of Congress Cataloging-in-Publication Data 97-71684
ISBN 978-0-615-64799-9

Dedicated to my mother and father whom I have grown to truly appreciate.

Also by Liz Koch

Books:
Core Awareness: Enhancing Yoga, Pilates, Exercise, & Dance
Maiden, Mother, Crone: Our Pleasure Playlist

Audio CDs:
Psoas & Back Pain
Unraveling Scoliosis

Articles:
Massage Magazine USA
The Iliopsoas Muscle: A Bio-Reverent Approach (Trauma) Part 1
The Iliopsoas Muscle: A Bio-Reverent Practical Approach (Trauma) Part 2

Midwifery Today USA
Birthing Fear: The Iliopsoas Muscle

The Doula USA
Intuitive Mothering
The Psoas Muscle During Pregnancy & Birth

Vegetarian Times & Connections USA
Your Back In Gardening

Yoga & Health UK
Core Awareness: 5 Most Important Things to Know about your Psoas Muscle
Gaining Flexible Hip Sockets
How to Help Children Develop Core Awareness & Avoid Chronic Pain
Illuminating The Iliacus
Sacred Sacrum

Yoga Journal USA
The Psoas Is...

What People are Saying about The Psoas Book

I just read The Psoas Book, *and I want you to know that you've helped me to change my life. The technique you presented helped release trapped emotions (fear). After doing the releasing exercise just once, I stood up and felt an amazing difference in my body.*
Athlete and personal fitness trainer for 14 years with a physical therapy background

I have read The Psoas Book *from cover to cover and it makes so much sense. This information is so helpful to my clients...they are really feeling the difference.*
Naturopath & Massage Therapist

I cannot tell you how much better I am because of what I learned from The Psoas Book *and the exercises... What you offer is so important!*
Pam England CNM,MA nurse/midwife

We LOVE the Psoas Book
Jivamukti Yoga Center, New York city

I have been practicing constructive rest position and am feeling some differences internally since recently reading The Psoas Book. *It helped me to understand why my body is so out of balance and I have not walked correctly for years.*
RN &, massage therapist

About 12 years ago, I found The Psoas Book *and was delighted to find at least one other person that is convinced that the Psoas is more than just a hip flexor muscle.*
Sue Hitzmann, Founder of MELT Method

The Psoas Book is the comprehensive guide on your journey toward knowing your psoas
Lene Guldbech Uttrup, Danish Psychomotor Therapist

I've spent thousands of dollars on chiropractors and physical therapists - asking for help with the chronic pain in my right hip. None have spoken about the psoas - that's the problem! Because of reading The Psoas Book *and my practicing the explorations, I can now walk without my right hip numbing out.*
Long distance runner

I have done yoga, pilates, been rolfed, had chiropractic treatments, physical therapy, myofacial release, and massages and was seriously considering looking into a hip replacement when I came across The Psoas Book.
Lbor and delivery nurse

The Psoas Book *is required reading for my Teaching, Terminology and Technique Classes*
Joanna Medl Shaw, Dance Instructor

What People are Saying about The Psoas Workshops

Liz provides this important muscle with an informed and experiential context that moves the mystique of the psoas into the realm of core experience and the opportunity for self-healing.
Ronnie Oliver, Aston-Patterning Practitioner & Advanced Instructor (San Francisco, CA)

The workshop was EXCELLENT. I've been practicing yoga for 22 years and teaching for 17. I came back... feeling compelled to rethink both my personal practice and my classes. I've been working from the outside without the monumental awareness of the core/psoas.
Workshop participant (Washington DC)

I golfed my best game ever this week I believe a relaxed Psoas had something to do with it!
Workshop participant (Santa Fe MN)

My teaching has changed, as I consider the Psoas throughout each session, I know each of my clients have benefited.
Pilates Instructor & workshop participant (Drysdale, Australia)

The workshop gave me an alternative model for looking at the body that returned a sense of wonder...
Pilates Instructor and workshop participant (Bristol, UK)

I think the biggest thing I got out of the workshop was to listen to myself and have more confidence in what I am doing.
Martial Arts student and workshop participant (Somerset, UK)

Deep gratitude to Liz Koch for creating the opportunity for us to bathe in the nourishment of the primordial waters of being.
Yoga teacher & workshop participant (Santa Monica, CA)

After 33 years of taking continuing education classes, I recently completed Liz Koch's Introductory Psoas workshop. I now realize that a working knowledge of the psoas- that is, how the psoas functions in human movement, the effects upon the body of chronic psoas tightness, and how to release that tightness-is an essential 'tool of the trade' for bodyworkers. I highly recommend this course and am sorry I did not take it many years ago. Another bonus to this course is the improvement in your own posture and ease of movement that you will experience if you use the information from the workshop to release, lengthen, and tone your own psoas.
Workshop Participant Marybetts Sinclair, LMT, author of Modern Hydrotherapy for the Massage Therapist, and Massage for Healthier Children, and Pediatric Massage Therapy.

Thanks for gracing Iowa with your presence and your profound knowledge of the psoas
Betsy Rippentrop PhD, Heartland Yoga, Instructor & Workshop participant (Iowa City)

What People are Saying about The Psoas Workshops

Liz Koch's insightful teachings solved a problem that had imprisoned my meditation practice for 30 years.

Workshop participant (Colorado)

I was very interested in iliopsoas and recognize that the iliopsoas plays a very important role in our life, emotion, activity, and health. But it was very mysterious for me. At the workshop I was strongly impressed by Liz Koch and her words..' juicy verses dry tissue'. Through the workshop I could understand more deeply.

Workshop participant (Japan)

I do believe you really are what you (Liz Koch) know, and that you practice what you preach. You were very fun to be around. You shared yourself by living in and through what you shared. I am charmed and honored to have been there.

Workshop Participant (Scotland, UK)

WOW, yoga went great tonight the day after the two-day workshop! Felt very fluid & loose.

Workshop participant

Thank you again for a great workshop. What I have learned and been able to utilize has transformed my life and work. I am eager to broaden my knowledge of the psoas and the mind/body/spirit/connection. My awareness of my body has changed dramatically.

Workshop participant

I loved your workshop - lots of good information for continued research and I really appreciate your encouragement to understand and explore the psoas work on an experiential level (not so easy but essential). More importantly though, I really liked working with you and hope to do further studies with you in the future. You are such a beautiful woman and I felt warmed by your softness and sensuality.

Workshop participant

I wanted to contact you and let you know how much I enjoyed the Psoas workshop.I've never experienced anything quite like I did last week. As a novice to the natural... type fields...it could have been overwhelming and frustrating at times but the wealth of information in that room was wonderful to absorb and I was honored to be a part of.

Workshop participant (New York)

Your work with the Psoas is a strong influence on my yoga teaching & teacher training.

Yoga Teacher & Workshop participant (UK)

What People are Saying about The Psoas Workshops

Your own enthusiasm and love for your work is inspirational and set an engaging energy into motion. The whole group was wonderful, open, attentive, and ready to share.

Workshop participant (New York)

You have convinced me that this 'misunderstood' and 'overworked' muscle holds the key not only to proper body alignment/posture but is the storehouse of our emotional health

Workshop participant (California)

Liz Koch is an exceptional healer, teacher, author, and expert on the psoas muscle. Her years of experience as a somatic educator and bodyworker and her natural intuition about the innate intelligence of the body makes her a very informative and insightful presenter. When I met her she was quite familiar with Ortho-Bionomy. ® Her training changed the way I work, bringing an increased focus on the importance of the psoas muscle and the means of releasing it. Her book and articles in various professional journals continually provide possibilities of working with the entire person.

Barry Krost Master Bodyworker (Ortho-Bionomy ®) & workshop participant (Chicago)

Your voice, and presentation facilitated the psoas explorations. I deepened into my core like never before...

Workshop participant (Ohio)

I was able to begin the process of 'juicing up my psoas" ~ if felt heavenly!

Workshop participant (Connecticut)

I wanted to share with you what one of the workshop attendees told me last year. She came up to me, very excited, and told me that what she learned in the workshop saved her from the knee surgery that she thought she might need.

Workshop participant (Nashville)

Thank you for opening me to an unexplored part of my body. I felt like I simultaneously accessed something very deep emotionally and barely touched the surface physically to something so integral to my being.

Workshop participant (Australia)

The Psoas Book & Workshop is must read for everyone who wishes to have a deep and conscious understanding of the psoas and its relationship to the body. This book amazes you over and over again. This muscle and its expression should not be underestimated. Read it, take the workshop, and feel the great understanding in your own body!

Workshop participant (Denmark)

"When one tugs at a single thing in nature,
he finds it attached to the rest of the world."

~John Muir

Contents

Preface: 30th Edition

The plethora of technological devices now available as well as the extraordinary response from my readers has inspired me to revitalize and upgrade The Psoas Book. I am delighted with this 30th Anniversary edition. Updating the manuscript and images has given me the opportunity to clarify my understanding of the psoas muscle and to elucidate my ideas for you, the reader.

This book has truly come full circle. Starting as a simple blue booklet, I wrote the first edition with neither a computer nor any layout alternative but to cut and paste on lineboard. Having no duplicate of the original and having my printer go out of business taking my originals, my second edition was a 'hodge-podge' of texts and salvaged images that were materialized on what then was my very first computer. Being a busy mom of three children and an international educator, I never imagined myself returning to reconstruct The Psoas Book. I aspired to move forward and spend my time with my family, teaching, and writing about Core Awareness. 30 years later, however, all of the generous appreciation and feedback has motivated me to create a well-written manuscript. Seeing as this is my fundamental book concerning the psoas, it deserves my full, unflagging attention.

The concept of the psoas has transformed into a family enterprise: my son, Adam, is my web designer for Core Awareness; my daughter, Megan, is currently apprenticing with my colleague Bob Cooley; and Lily, my daughter and editor, is a ferocious writer whose skill and love have supported my ability to fully articulate my ideas. This edition is both a celebration of a book for which I can be proud of and a celebration of my family and life.

~Liz Koch [California 2012]

Preface: 1st Edition

The material presented in this book has been collected over the past seven years with the intention of offering it to students who have requested reading material and information concerning the psoas muscle. The knowledge provided in this book is information that I have found most helpful in my search for balanced posture.

I have a history of scoliosis (spinal curvature), muscle spasms, a limited range of movement, and physical awkwardness, which I assumed I would live with and work around for the rest of my life. It was not until I was in my twenties when an introduction to yoga opened me to the possibilities of experiencing my body differently. It was a powerful experience and I attempted to continue along those lines. Finding it too difficult to work alone, I sought and found my first teacher and beloved friend, Robert Cooley. I worked with Bob for three years at his Boston school, The Moving Center, Inc. Originally a dancer, Bob became interested in why dancers easily injure themselves. The more he learned, the more he seemed to move away from dance (though he loves dancing) and developed a more specific interest in movement. As Bob's perceptive eye and keen sense of movement grew more experienced, he taught me what he knew, encouraging me to learn to sense my own body while developing an eye for seeing the human body in motion.

While Bob was investing his time and effort in releasing and lengthening his psoas, I spent the first six months that I worked with him just trying to find out what I was looking for and where it was in my body. It took a long time to realize how subtle and deep the sensation of the psoas could be. At first, I felt miles way from myself. However, as I worked quietly, with Bob's encouragement and humor, I learned the value of directing my attention toward sensation.

I found the territory to be unknown, often scary, and sometimes it felt all too personal. Yet being in that warm sunlit room, surrounded by green plants, oriental carpets, and friendly people, I allowed myself the time and opportunity to venture inside and look around. We were all trying in similar ways to speak of what we were sensing: "I sense my psoas on the left side and it is more contracted than on the right. Now, I sense it stretching. I sense a quivering around my rib cage and a sensation of heat moving into my legs...." We followed our attention as it moved through the body. Later, it was fun trying to catch an emotion or a thought as it flew by connected to a sensation like a tail on a kite: "I have an ache sensation in my right hip socket, I notice a feeling of frustration and anger....an image of my father comes up. I think I would like to kick him...." And then laughter - a sense of humor toward my conditioning was being cultivated.

When I left Boston for out west I was both ready and scared. I wondered what would happen without the support and understanding of Bob and the studio. Once settled in California, I began again on my own. Eventually, I had the idea to try to gather other people to work with me. I wrote Bob at the same time that he wrote to me suggesting that I start a class. And so I did. Four years went by as I continued to learn from teaching. Staying one step ahead of my students, I often felt that I was being pushed by the class rather than leading it. Through teaching and studying, I explored various methods as I searched for a better understanding of the process occurring under my nose.

I met my acupressure teacher, Aminah Raheem, in Santa Cruz a year after I began to teach and became interested in Jin Shin Do, a gentle meditative form of Japanese acupressure based on the Chinese meridian point system. Inspired, I became certified as a practitioner. Practicing Jin Shin Do illuminated to me a whole new way of perceiving the body, and this different perspective influenced my approach to teaching "Postural Transformation."

I was not very touched by most of the methods I encountered, although I appreciated certain aspects of them, until a birthday present gave me an opportunity to experience Aston-Patterning an approach developed by Judith Aston to free the body of unnecessary stress both structurally and in everyday movement. Generally speaking, I had approached my body directly - I worked through my own awareness rather than

Preface: 1st Edition

seeking people to 'work on me.' In fact, I felt especially offended when anyone wanted to try to correct my posture. For me, body work was a tool to develop my sensitivity and to increase my awareness; any postural change was a bonus. I was, however, moved by the work with Ronnie Neufeld-Oliver, a masseuse and Aston-Patterning teacher. She was equally interested in acupressure, which gave us a unique opportunity to experience each other's way of working, to exchange ideas, and to develop a close friendship.

Aston-Patterning responded to a question I had begun to formulate concerning the need for an organized way of approaching the body. I was not sure yet what I meant by that, but I sensed that Bob's work was not yet formed into a method. I found that Aston-Patterning responded to my need not by imposing an image of the right posture on my body, but by evoking my body's natural ability to organize, balance, and coordinate itself. I also liked the method because it worked not only with releasing the psoas, but also with engaging it in movement. For the first time, I experienced volume, depth, and a three-dimensional quality to my body. My scoliosis began unraveling, which shed light on its emotional and attitudinal components. This might be considered a miracle compared to the standard approach to scoliosis, which includes stringent exercise, back braces, drugs, body casts, and vertebrae fusing. With Aston-Patterning, each step led to the next, so that in a manner of speaking, the work was always digestible. I now feel as though an elaborate three-dimensional mosaic pattern is being constructed. The further I go toward sensing myself, the more I find that my body opens to receive and experience life.

Although this booklet focuses on only one aspect of the body, the psoas muscle, I think it is impossible to separate one element from the whole. Therefore, I suggest that anyone pursuing an understanding of his or her body try to perceive and work with the body as an integrated whole: as a receiver, transformer, and transmitter of substances or energies, which function as part of a larger universal body and that demands our attention, sensitivity, and respect.

~Liz Koch [California, 1981]

Preface: 2nd Edition

What began as a simple student manual grew over the years to be a layperson's and professional's guide to the iliopsoas muscle. I have worked with the psoas muscle for over 20 years and still find it an intriguing subject. The psoas represents the deepest, instinctual qualities of energy in the human being. It is from the area of the psoas that wise women and wise men ground themselves. With an integrated, well functioning psoas comes a quiet safe haven to move from and be within. The image that appears for me is a tribal image: a wise bushman whose instinctual self has transcended survival skills to the 'fine art of being' on Mother Earth. From this deeply grounded, stable place we allow the heart and mind to soar. Only when the psoas is free to move, can the energy of our body flow smoothly, our emotions balance, and our thoughts become integrated.

I would like to acknowledge all the people who made this second edition possible. My son, Adam, who taught me to use a computer and who has served as my computer graphics technician; my husband, Jeff Oberdorfer, and my two daughters, Megan and Lily, who 'put up' with my constant dialogue about the psoas muscle; Victor Collins D.C., who has served as both healer and teacher, thank you for helping me articulate my ideas as well as my own psoas muscle; my colleague, Ronnie Oliver, who continues to be my best friend and with whom I love sharing ideas and combining our teaching skills; and Bob Cooley without whom I might never have discovered I had a psoas muscle. He is still my teacher, good friend, and greatest supporter of my work. Last but not least, I thank all my students who keep asking me questions for which I do not have the answer.

~Liz Koch [California, 1997]

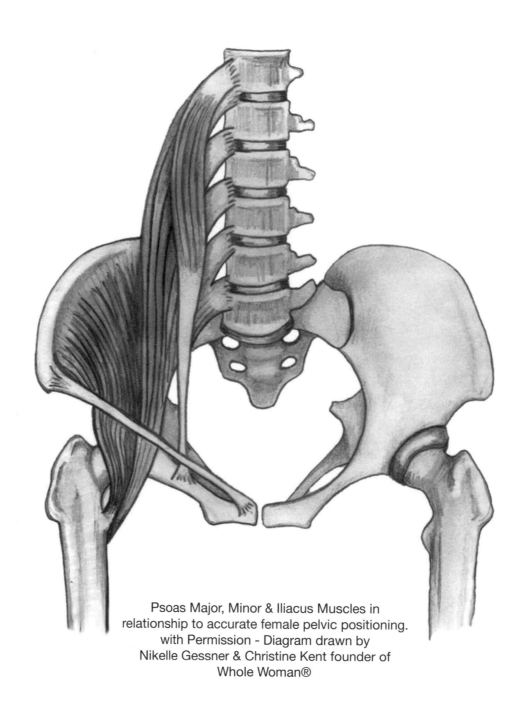

Psoas Major, Minor & Iliacus Muscles in
relationship to accurate female pelvic positioning.
with Permission - Diagram drawn by
Nikelle Gessner & Christine Kent founder of
Whole Woman®

Chapter 1: Location

The psoas muscle (pronounced so-az) is the keystone of a balanced, well-organized body. It is a massive muscle, approximately 16 inches long that directly links the spine to the legs. There are two psoas muscles, one emerging from each side of the lumbar spine. Anatomically each consists of a psoas major and a psoas minor. The psoas major has its origin on the side of the spinal vertebrae and the transverse processes. It emerges at the level of the twelfth thoracic vertebra (T12) and from each of the five lumbar vertebrae (L1-5).

The psoas minor is a vanishing muscle. It originates at T12 and grows into a thin tendon at the pelvic rim. A relic of the human organism's primordial ancestry, it is thought to be a disappearing muscle as the body evolves from a semi-flexed to an upright being. It is possible to have only one psoas minor or none at all.

When referring to the psoas muscle, this book is addressing the psoas major because it is the predominant aspect of the muscle. The psoas major may vary, growing out from T12 or out from the lumbar vertebra (L1). The psoas major (psoas) traverses from the spine, through the pelvic basin, over the ball and socket hip joints, into the lesser trochanter of the femur bones.

The psoas does not attach directly to the pelvic basin, but indirectly influences the pelvis through its relationship with the ribcage and femurs. More specifically, the psoas influences the pelvic basin as it shares a common tendon at the lesser trochanter with the iliacus muscle.

Location

The iliacus is a fan-shaped muscle lining each ilium of the inside of the pelvic basin. When spoken of together, the iliacus and psoas are referred to as the iliopsoas complex. The iliopsoas complex directly influences abdominal organ functioning, viscera, nerves, and the skeletal balance of the pelvic basin. The health of both the psoas and the iliacus are interdependent upon one another because of their common tendon. What transpires in one muscle will be reflected within the other.

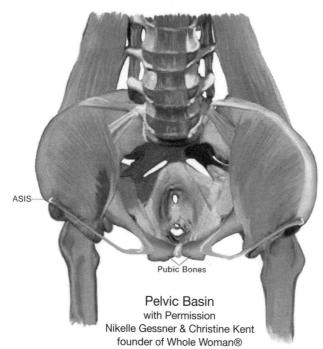

ASIS

Pubic Bones

Pelvic Basin
with Permission
Nikelle Gessner & Christine Kent
founder of Whole Woman®

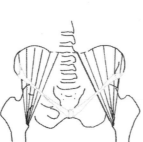

Outline of the Fan Shaped
Iliacus Muscle

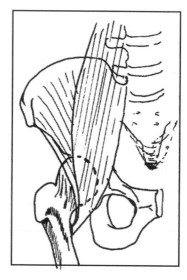

The Iliopsoas Complex

Location

The psoas is located at the central axis (core) of the human body. It grows directly out of the thoracic and lumbar vertebrae (or spine). Although there is a common perception that a muscularly rigid core is analogous with a strong core, and that muscles hold the body up against the powerful force of gravity, it is actually the spinal vertebra's weight-bearing capacity that results in a healthy, powerful, and resilient core. Ultimately what allows the spinal vertebrae to bear weight efficiently is a supple, dynamic, and responsive psoas.

The knobby projections that can be felt along the back of the spine may lead to the belief that the spinal column is located in the back of the body. However, what is actually felt when a person touches his or her back is the transverse processes, which are wing-like protrusions extending out from the spine. The spinal column vertebrae, encasing the spinal cord, is deeply set and occupies approximately one-half of the diameter of the body from the front to the back. This central position and its subtle triangular shape, along with its bilateral symmetry, gives the spine its immense power. Additionally, the S-shaped curve configuration of the spinal column provides resiliency in its dynamic response to gravity. Hence all movement, power, expression, and support manifests directly from the physical core of the located at the central axis.

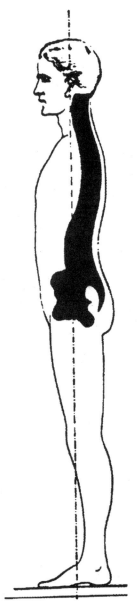

Central Axis

Location

Another common misconception is the location of the hip sockets. When asked where the hip sockets are, most people will point to the sides of their hips because that is where movement is most often experienced when the leg is in action. In reality, the side of the hip is accurately the location of the greater trochanter an aspect of the femur. The actual ball and socket hip joint is located in the front of the pelvis where the socket of the pelvis and the ball of the femur join together. Here is where the core pelvic basin and the femur bone (upper leg) meet and create a joint, which articulates so that movement transpires.

It is also here at the ball and socket hip joints (hip sockets), where weight through the pelvis transfers from the center axis (spine) into the two legs and feet. The fact that the psoas passes directly over the ball and socket hip joint and grows into the lessor trochanter, directly affects the articulation and range of motion within the hip sockets and each leg.

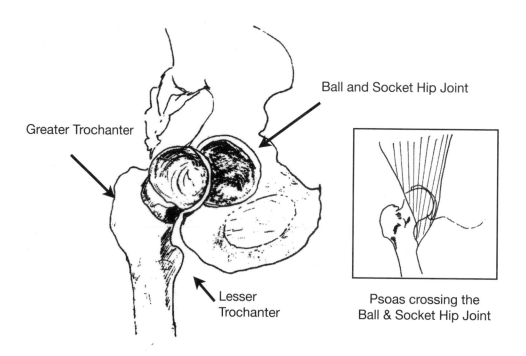

Greater Trochanter

Ball and Socket Hip Joint

Lesser Trochanter

Psoas crossing the Ball & Socket Hip Joint

Location

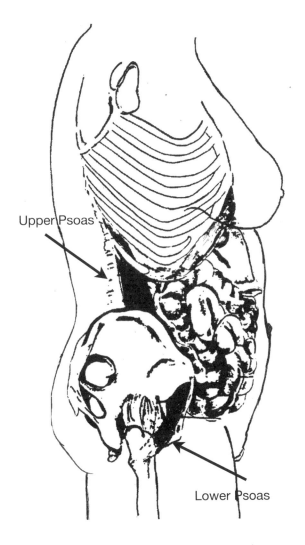

Upper Psoas

Lower Psoas

Diagonal Psoatic Shelf

The shape and breadth of the psoas is multidirectional. The psoas, approximately the thickness of a human fist, moves in an oblique plane from deep within the solar plexus, located at T12, and surfaces over the ball and socket hip joint to then traverse back toward the lessor trochanter of the upper medial femur. It spreads laterally as it diagonally traverses through the pelvic cavity creating a "psoatic shelf." The psoatic shelf provides a muscular support for all the abdominal organs, which are superficial to (above) the psoas. The psoas is deepest at the solar plexus, which is the location of the spine at the level of T12 and it is most superficial (comes to the surface of the body) as it crosses over the ball and socket hip joint.

Location

Having a clear image of the layered leg muscles that surround the femur and the pelvic basin is helpful in understanding how deep the psoas truly is especially in comparison to the superficial quadricep muscles. The psoas is located at the skeletal level of the femur bone; with the majority of thigh and leg muscles superficial to the psoas.

The location of the psoas as central within the human core cannot be complete without including the muscles of the upper body, specifically the trapezius muscle.

The massive diamond-shaped trapezius grows upwards toward the skull beginning its journey at the back of the dorsal twelfth thoracic vertebra (T12). On the ventral side of the same vertebra at the solar plexus, the psoas muscle begins its journey down, also forming a triangle, toward both legs.

Known as the lumbodorsal junction, T12 is a vitally important vertebra where two very powerful muscles emerge at two different layers of depth, to move in two opposite directions.

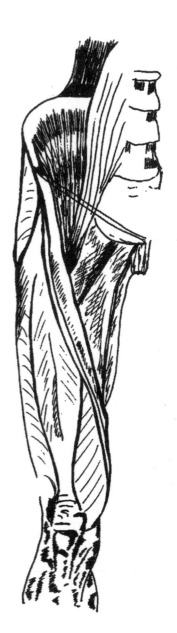

Leg/Hip Muscles - Front View

Location

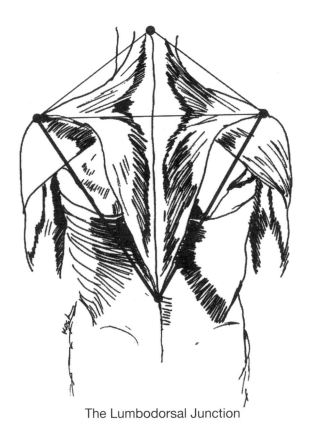

The Lumbodorsal Junction

At the lumbodorsal junction, resides not only the trapezius, psoas, and solar plexus but the respiratory diaphragm, a lordotic muscle similar to a jellyfish that opens and closes moving through the cavity of the trunk. The diaphragm is not generally experienced as part of the lumbar musculature, and yet its origin emerges deep from within the 4th and 5th vertebrae of the lumbar spine. The diaphragm is a muscular and tendinous structure separating the chest from the abdomen. The diaphragm forms the floor for the thoracic cage with the heart above it and a roof for the abdominal cavity with the liver, gallbladder, stomach, and spleen beneath its domelike surface.

The dome shaped diaphragm's undulating expansive movement massages not only the organs, but the vertebrae stimulating synovial fluid along the spine to the brain. Intimately interacting with the psoas, the diaphragm's central position makes it responsive to and influenced by multiple rhythms of the body.

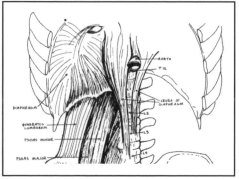

Diaphragm

The esophagus penetrates through the diaphragm and the major aorta of the heart flows just behind it. Both the psoas and the aorta move through the core and following each other , both pass over the ball and socket hip joints of the pelvis. The aorta, having already split into two arteries just below the navel, moves through on its journey to the legs and the feet.

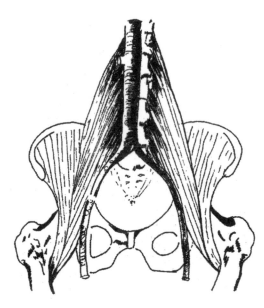

Path of Major Aorta & Psoas

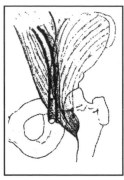

Artery Crossing
at Hip Socket

Location

The lumbar nerve plexus is a complex network of nerves adjacent to the psoas. The nerve ganglia of the lumbar is known as the abdominal, gut, or enteric brain. The psoas is involved in a complex communication amongst the organs and viscera as well as the central, autonomic, and enteric nervous systems. The psoas resides where gut feelings may be sensed. The upper psoas and diaphragm are located at a locus known as the solar plexus. An energetic center for personal power, the solar plexus is where unwanted or overwhelming emotions are attempted to be controlled. Ida Rolf in her book, *Rolfing: The Integration of the Human Structure*, explains that:

> Along the anterior lateral surface of the entire spine lies the sympathetic trunk of the autonomic nervous system... This more archaic nerve unit is thought to be at a level below our voluntary control, although recent findings shed a certain doubt on this. It forms a series of ganglia that are centers integrating associated nerve elements. The great solar plexus, locus of the largest of these, is sometimes called the abdominal brain. It lies approximately at the level where the psoas and diaphragm juxtapose. The lumbar plexus, with its network for visceral and muscular intercommunication, is the next lower neighbor and is embedded in the surface of the psoas itself.[1]

The kidneys float directly above each psoas and the nerves traveling to and from the reproductive organs embed through the psoas. The vital location and interrelationship of the psoas with the diaphragm, organs, blood, and nerves is what gives the psoas its powerful unifying function.

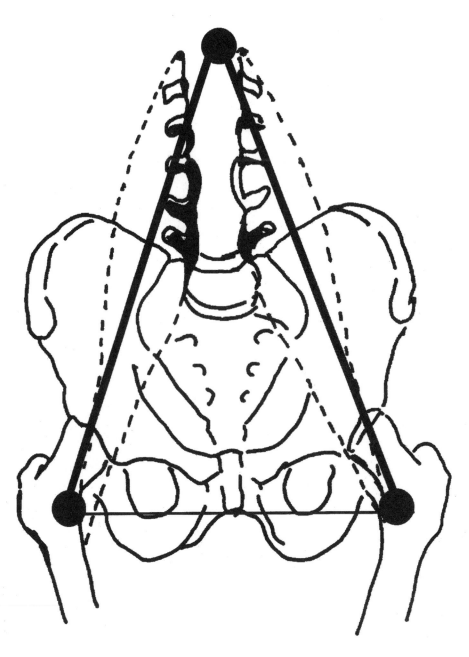

Solar Plexus & Psoas
Energetic Triangle

Chapter 2: Function

The psoas is a multi-joint muscle emerging out of six joints and passing over two. The psoas can tense and shorten as well as expand and lengthen in sections depending upon the work being required of it and the neuromuscular habits of a person. The psoas is bio-mechanically defined as a hip flexor; however, in reality it is a pendulum supporting the free swing of the leg while walking.

As a pendulum, the movement of the psoas stimulates the flow of fluids throughout tissue and cells. In normal walking, the psoas is expressive: toning and lengthening with every step. In a normal range of motion, its action stimulates the viscera and massages the spine (core). When able to move freely, rather than be used as a structural support, the supple expressive psoas and lumbar plexus is a source of the energy for animating the legs, and plays a focal role in activating both sexual and anal functions.

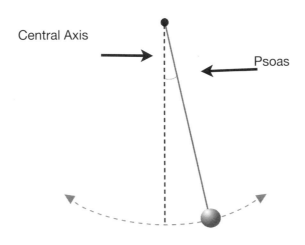

Central Axis

Psoas

Free Swing of the Leg in Motion

Along with the psoas, the iliacus and obturator (small intrinsic muscles located within the pelvic basin) create a dynamic balanced pelvis that is free-swinging, providing freedom of movement through the legs and feet. In *Rolfing: The Integration of the Human Structure,* Rolf describes the importance of the psoas in relationship to walking: "Sturdy, balanced walking (in which the leg is flexed through activation of the psoas, not of the rectus femoris) thus involves the entire body at its core level."[2] This exemplifies how walking is a movement that is initiated not in the leg muscles but is animated from within the core and is carried by the psoas through the leg and foot.

The psoas and the erector spinae muscles have a reciprocal and balancing relationship. Running along the posterior spine, the erector spinae muscles are often considered 'weak.' However, it is when the upper psoas muscle is supple and at full length that the erector spinae regain their tone.

The psoas also functions as a counterbalance to the rector abdominal muscle, maintaing a centered front-back (anterior-posterior) relationship. However the abdominals muscles are directly balanced by the length of the hamstring muscles located on the back of leg and tuberosities (sits bones).

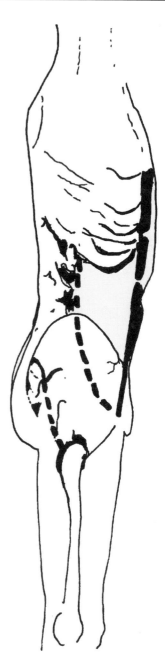

Functional Psoas

Function

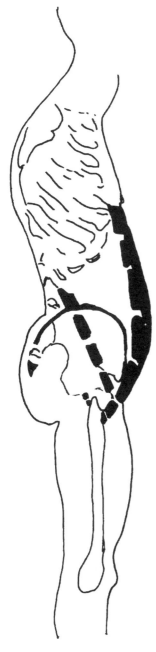

Shortened Psoas

The balance between the iliopsoas complex, the rector abdominal muscles, and the hamstring muscles helps to bring a sense of wholeness and a functional relationship to the core. The lack of this relationship often leads to what author Karlfried Graf Von Durkheim terms as a "chest out–belly in" posture. In his book, *Hara: The Vital Centre Of Man*, Durkheim writes how the chest out–belly in posture "misses the natural structure of the human body." He illuminates that when the center of gravity shifts upward toward the chest it "forces a man to swing between hypertension and slackness."[3]

It may be no surprise that fitness and exercise programs offered in today's Western culture focuses so intensely and invest so much time and money on isolating and strengthening the superficial abdominal muscles. Lost is a much deeper sense and level of kinesthetic knowing found only within the belly core. Exercises such as sit-ups and push-ups cannot only exhaust the psoas, but also can provoke additional tension along an already strained and constricted core. This stress only decreases efficiency and motility while further burdening a person who already lacks the support and nourishment necessary for dwelling deep within the quieter aspects of his or her the core.

Function

A similar dynamic gets ignited if the psoas is misused as a hip flexor. Lost is the profound sense of neutrality found deep within the dynamic supple psoas. The natural harmony and rhythm of the core pendulum is disrupted, while the person experiences additional tension and pain within the ball and socket hip joint.

The vitality of the psoas depends upon how it is used or misused. The length and the breadth of the psoatic shelf will determine how all the abdominal organs rest within the pelvic basin. Only when the psoatic shelf is supple can it fully massage all the organs. However, if the psoas is engaged as a tensile structure, it will function as a 'guide wire' for stabilizing the spine. Picture a circus tent or bridge with its main pole and guy-wires stabilizing the structure. Similar to the tension cables that support the main pole, the psoas supports the spine by responding to any core disruption. Performing as a ligament, the psoas will eventually shorten and dry. The priority of the psoas is not to support, but to inform. As part of the fluid sympathetic neuro-core, the psoas is neutral, supple, and expressive.

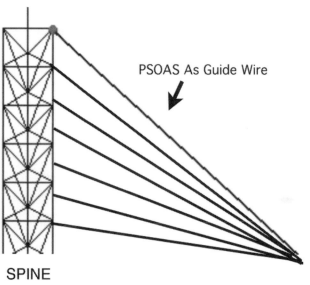

PSOAS As Guide Wire

SPINE

Chapter 3: Influence

Before delving into the nuances of the psoas and the various influences it has concerning the human being, there are a few basic concepts that need to be taken into consideration.

Firstly, the bones are focal to understanding the psoas. Simply put, bones support weight by responding to gravity. When the muscles support weight, rather than the bones bearing weight, it further disrupts the core and the muscle's ability to move the bones freely, resulting in continued muscular fatigue. More importantly, the misuse of muscles can disrupt proprioception, which is essential for skeletal alignment, equilibrium, flow, and orientation in time and space. Overdeveloped muscles can distort the shape of the bones, disrupt efferent and afferent nerve signals, and decrease blood circulation in and around the surrounding tissue, ligaments, and joints.[4] Awakening the bones and becoming skeletally aware is essential for being moved from the core.

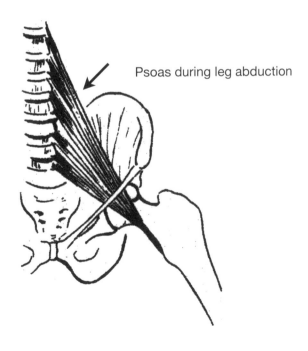

Psoas during leg abduction

Influence

For the joints to properly transfer weight and the functional psoas not to be misused as a support, it is crucial for the bones to be aligned. This alignment results in an energetic transmission that links the bones together creating a coherent skeletal system. Therefore, support is not achieved by muscular holding, but a relationship sensed within and throughout bone, ground, and gravity. Now, support can be experienced as subtle energy freely moving, without obstruction, throughout the body and linked by the joints like pearls on a string. The psoas influences and is influenced by this relationship between healthy functional joints as they transfer weight along the bones. Whether intentionally or unintentionally, enlisting the psoas for support ultimately determines the quality of skeletal coherency, the vitality of the psoas, as well as the postural stance of the person.

A shortened psoas is most often the result of continual misuse or disruption of skeletal coherency. A shortened psoas, visually seen as a forward thrusting pelvis, creates rotational differences in the spinal vertebrae, pelvic basin, legs, and feet. These distortions may express themselves as exaggerated curves in the lumbar, thoracic, and cervical spine. In the pelvis, a shortened psoas results in forward thrusts, lateral tilts, and twists. In the femurs, the result of a shortened psoas includes constricted movement in the ball and socket joint and distortions in lateral and medial rotation. Thus, when the psoas shortens, the relationship between bones continues to be fragmented giving the body a disjointed and disconnected appearance.

The difference between each psoas muscle also affects posture and range of motion. If the psoas is shorter on one side it may cause leg length discrepancies. Putting a lift in one shoe to compensate for this condition does not address the real problem. To have a healthy core, balancing the pelvic basin, articulating the joints, and increasing proprioception along with the releasing and lengthening of the psoas must all be addressed.

Why the psoas shortens more on one side than the other is a question with an answer that leads to a new perspective concerning the human body in motion. Attempting to just balance the two psoas muscles to correct this disparity is not enough to resolve the problem. The psoas may be shorter on one side due to an injury that has resulted in exaggerated patterns of compensation, a continual stress such as carrying a heavy bag on one shoulder, organ functioning, or emotional expression due to a person's unique pattern of holding tension. Whatever the reason, rather than evaluate the body as a static object, the body must be perceived as a living process. Only then can the core be understood as a continual expression of both internal and external forces. The human body is a 360 degree organism that is shaped by biological, social, and environmental influences, which manifest in 3-dimensional spirals.

The spiral is a natural pattern of nature. Look at the whorls of human fingertips, the shells on the beach, the pinecones, plants, and ferns of the forest, all of these spiral patterns are shaped by the spinning earth. Water spirals down the drain and the hair on the human head is borne out of a swirl. Moreover, through a microscope spirals can be seen flowing in the helical structure of DNA and through a telescope the galaxies can be seen flowing in cosmic spirals. Consequently, working with spirals engenders the need to explore strategies for unravelling. To resolve and elicit harmony in the core involves unraveling patterns of tension not simply straightening a person out, in order to nourish the whole person's sense of integrity.[5]

Influence

Not only is a person's body not a static form, but also it is not linear or symmetrical. Bodies are complex, fluid, bilateral beings and although symmetrical movement can be seen in very young children when learning to walk, this movement quickly complexifies: progressing from symmetrical into diagonal (spiral) patterns as the child's neuromuscular system matures. In her article, "*Inherent Movement Patterns In Man*," author Susan Campbell explains walking and running as a symmetrical-to-diagonal movement progression:

> The first few independent steps of the infant are usually taken with the arms raised in a protective symmetrical position and the legs advance in a primitive external rotation-abduction pattern. The wide base of support in the early stages of walking demonstrates the unreliability of equilibrium reaction at this age.[6]

Thus, as a child matures, the pattern moves toward an asymmetrical diagonal pattern. The wide base of support closes and "In contrast, the confident toddler demonstrates arm swings which are reciprocally patterned with leg movements, narrowed bases of support and leg patterns which are spiral and diagonal in direction."[7] Returning to these early developmental cross patterning explorations can help to improve motor skills and increase skeletal proprioception. Doing so helps to nourish the psoas as well as avoid injury, which is one of the leading cause of an overused psoas.

Although overuse of the psoas can be due to faulty posture, the fundamental cause is a lack of developmental proprioception that creates this faulty way of moving, which then can eventually lead to low back, neck, and knee injuries.

Influence

When the psoas is overused due to a lack of proprioception, it eventually loses its healthy, dynamic expression. Caught up in a lack of safety and support, the psoas communicates this disruption loud and clear. By compensating for the lack of skeletal support, over time the psoas dries, shortens, and becomes constricted.

The dry, shortened psoas perpetuates poor skeletal positioning. If the excursion length of the psoas (the length of the muscle in movement) does not allow the bones to be free to move in response to gravity, maintaining accurate positioning or executing movement is curtailed. This invariably results in further substitution of other muscles and exacerbates muscle strain, exhaustion, and overall tension.

If the "resting length" (the ideal length of a muscle when neither stretching nor contracting) of the psoas has shortened, it will pull on the pelvis, strain the back muscles, and close the spacial dimension of the ball and socket hip joint. When the pelvic hip sockets are constricted, the pelvis and leg move as a unit rather than as an articulated joint. Instead of rotation occurring at the round head of the femur, which moves within the cup-shaped ilium, or the pelvis rolling around the head of the femur ball, rotation stops at the joint and occurs by twisting at the knees and/or low spine (L 4 and L 5).

Whether the psoas shortens and dries due to its compensation or is intentionally engaged for additional muscular support, any constriction in the psoas will thrust the ribcage forward encouraging thoracic rather than abdominal breathing. Pulled forward and down, the ribcage limits the diaphragm from fully descending and therefore its range of motion is lost. When the diaphragm can no longer fulfill its function of stimulating and massaging the organs, nerves, and blood, circulation may be impaired.

By pushing the diaphragm forward in space, the constricted psoas impedes upon the esophagus as it penetrates through the diaphragm traveling to the stomach. The major aorta, which is juxtaposed with the diaphragm, may also be curtailed due to a constricted upper psoas. Because the aorta flows directly over the ball and socket hip joint, the psoas can block circulation as the aorta travels to the legs and feet.

A dry, constricted psoas will compress the torso influencing the structural positioning of the bones and lessening the internal space available for the organs and viscera. For example, digestion, assimilation, and basic elimination, may be disturbed due to a constricted lumbar plexus.[8] When the psoas muscle is engaged improperly, every aspect of the metabolic process may suffer.

Whether or not the autonomic ganglia and lumbar plexus are able to do their job effectively influences adrenal and kidney health and therefore a person's immune system. The kidneys float directly above the psoas muscle and thus depend upon a supple, functional psoas. When the psoas is dry and constricted, the fluidity of the kidneys may be adversely impacted.

The constricted psoas also influences the reproductive system. The nerves going to the uterus and ovaries directly penetrate the psoas. When the psoas is dry and shortened, it can both compress nerves and limit space in the pelvic basin, which can reposition the organs. For many women, menstrual cramps are not the result of cramping inside the uterus, but are caused by a constricted psoas. When women are taught to release the psoas muscle, they often

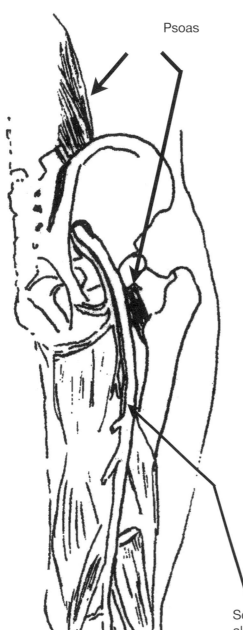

Psoas

Sciatic Nerve
along the back of pelvis and leg

experience relief from cramping and low back pain (see Chapter 8).

Sciatic pain, a condition involving the major nerve running through the pelvis and down the back of the leg, may also be caused and/or relieved by the health of the iliopsoas complex. When the psoas is constricted and the pelvis tilts forward, the sciatic notch, through which the sciatic nerve passes, can impinge upon the nerve. Irritated, the impingement can cause pain in the buttocks as well as down the side and back of the leg. By fanning open the iliacus, releasing the psoas, and toning the outward rotators (while balancing the pelvis), sciatic pain can be resolved. Furthermore, scoliosis, kyphosis, and other structural problems may all be approached, improved, and resolved by working with the psoas.

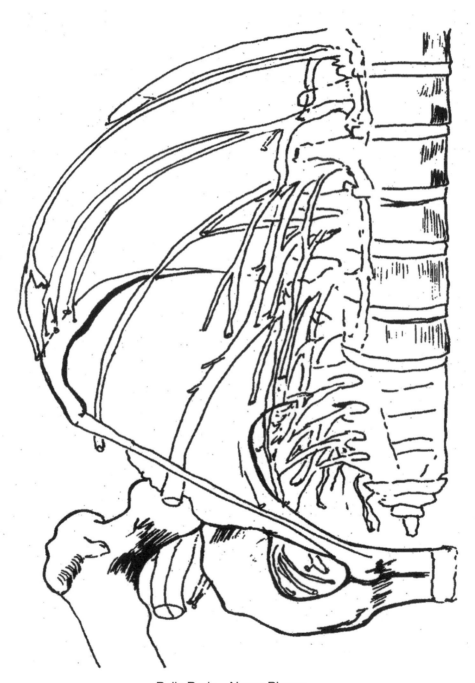

Belly Brain - Nerve Plexus

Chapter 4: Fear Response

There is only one expression of fear that is considered instinctive and not dependent upon personal experience: the fear of falling. The fear (or startle) response occurs through a complex set of nerve impulses in reaction to a sudden loss of support. The psoas, a part of the fear response, is called into action rolling the midline into a fetal curl.

The sense of falling registers in the vestibular apparatus located in the inner ear. The vestibular system contributes to the sense of balance and is responsible for spatial orientation, motility, and equilibrium. Being in close proximity to the cochlea (hearing) any intense excitation occurring in the auditory system can stimulate the vestibular system. After the first three weeks of life, when the infant's hearing is more developed, loud noises can stimulate and set off not only the fear response, but also the infantile moro reflex. The fear response as well as the moro reflex can be observed in newborns and is regarded as an early form of defense and protection.

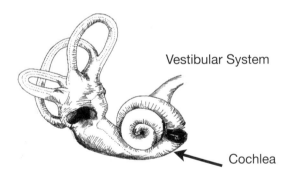

Vestibular System

Cochlea

An infant 'startles' when sensing a loss of support, reaching out to grab hold of the mother, this primal response helps to prevent falling. When protection is not reestablished, a second primal response, the fetal-curl, prepares the infant for falling, or to freeze and/or to 'play dead.'

Fear Response

In his book *Body & Mature Behavior*, Moshe Feldenkrais explains:

> One would expect the first reaction to be such as to withdraw the animal from danger as quickly as possible. It is not so when the frightening stimulus is too near or too violent. The first reaction to the frightening stimulus is a violent contraction of all the flexor muscles, especially of the abdominal region, a halt in breathing, soon followed by a whole series of vasomotor disturbances such as accelerated pulse, sweating, up to micturition and defecation....The initial flexor contraction.... [this] enables the animal to freeze and simulate death if the danger is too near.[9]

Fear is the only instinct that has the power to immobilize. Thus, it is no surprise that the core muscle, the psoas, plays an important role in the survival response of the organism: the flight-fight-freeze response. Perhaps it is the psoas that provides the fear response its power to literally stop a person in his or her tracks. Considered an involuntary muscle, the psoas cannot therefore consciously be controlled. However, the psoas is a primal messenger of core integrity, survival, and informs a person when he or she is safe or in danger.

When fetal curl is activated, the psoas (along with the flexor muscles) neurologically fires bringing the extremities together into a fetal-c curve. This creates a sense of safety while protecting the soft, vulnerable parts of the body: the vital organs, the genitals, and the head with the sensory receptors, the eyes, ears, nose, and mouth. The fear response curls the spine providing more resiliency when falling and protection against possible blows.

The whole being is involved when preparing for the flight-fight-freeze response. As adrenaline is released and the pulse accelerates, the startle response, or 'warding off,' expands the whole body by activating the extensor muscles in preparation for dynamic movement. The response fulfills itself through the action of running (flight) or warding off and standing ones ground (fight).

However, when the fear response fires repeatedly with little or no recovery time, this behavior conditions the body for its next attack by maintaining a state of perpetual tension. Because the organism no longer has the opportunity to return to a normal state of functioning, nourishment is diminished while the level of tension accumulates. This tension is experienced as anxiety. As the excitation builds, it radiates throughout the organs and nervous system. Moshe Feldenkrais elucidates:

> Fear and anxiety are here seen to be the sensation of impulses arriving at the central nervous system from the organs and viscera. There is ground for considering all emotions as excitations arising from the vegetative or autonomic nervous system and the organs, muscles, etc., that it innervates. The arrival of such impulses to the higher centres of the central nervous system is sensed as emotion.[10]

When the child, and later the adult, is unable to defend him or herself by fighting or fleeing from an overwhelming, unsafe, or terrifying situation, his or her only escape may be to disassociate. The fight-or-flight response or stress response entails the release of chemicals through a combination of nerve and hormonal signals that not only include cortisol and adrenaline but may also release natural opiates. Not only can a person go into physical shock, but he or she can also experience hyperarousal, which can than lead to psychically 'shutting down' by way of disassociating from what is or may be perceived to be a life-threatening situation. By shutting down or cutting off sensory input, a person disconnects from the present moment and thus numbs his or her pain.

Dissociating is a survival response. Although imagination and fantasy are focal facets of a person's ability to be creative and conceptualize, when utilized as a tool for dissociation, imagination and fantasy can desensitize and become a form of escape. Imagining that a painful situation is not occurring does not biologically satiate or exhaust the fear response. Instead it disconnects a person from the immediacy of sensation with the result being a diminished awareness. Although dissociation may be the only survival mechanism for a child in a potentially abusive situation, the psychic price is high because a deep sense of self is lost.

Although numb to sensation, the excitation continues inundating the system so that and the smallest reminder, such as an image, thought, or sound, can elicit a sense of fear or nameless anxiety. This pattern can become a reenactment as a person strives to avoid the organism's self-regulating attempt to reclaim balance.

People do not have 'weak' psoas muscles that need strengthening through standard muscle protocols, they have exhausted psoas muscles often due to an overwhelmed nervous system. The exhausted muscle is only thought to be weak because it behaves unresponsively. Eventually shortening, the exhausted psoas influences the breath, organs, and nervous system. The shortened psoas now becomes a part of the reenactment through its dryness and lack of vitality, which triggers a continual sense of anxiety and fear. If, however, a person consciously experiences and acknowledges sensations, it can ultimately motivate him or her to take action toward recovery, resolution, and the creation of a healthy life.

Even though humans have the ability to imagine and fantasize, what gives an image or thought its life, however, is the actual nerve excitation within the body. Thus, fear and trauma is biological not psychological. Fear literally vibrates through the nervous system and stirs the blood. No matter how subtle an experience may be, when a person is afraid, he or she may naturally attempt to control the unpleasant feelings by holding the breath and by increasing muscular tension. These methods of control result in the formation of layers of muscular rigidity known as muscular armoring.

Although Western thinking compartmentalizes sensations from feelings and thoughts, the organism is one whole being. Patterns of holding tension appear within the body through not only expressions of stance, but also through a person's receptivity, and attitude. Because muscular contractions are mostly voluntary (a person can control whether or not he or she contracts a muscle) stopping strong excitation is a very empowering feeling. Rather than feeling out of control or overwhelmed, a person's ability to flex his or her muscles can limit or even stop the intensity of sensation and feeling. Even though a person can build muscular armoring, the psoas, not being a voluntary muscle, cannot be controlled, it can only be surrounded by muscular girdling or armor. The psoas, therefore is directly expressive of how a person truly feels, without any defensiveness, deep within the core of his or her being.

For a young child, muscular control is often the only means of feeling safe. By abating feelings and sensations of anxiety, a child begins to get a handle on his or her emotions. When a child's feelings are habitually unacknowledged and problem-solving skills are lacking, a child will choose whatever physical attitude works best to bring his or her feelings and sensations under control. Feldenkrais notes: "passive safety is brought about by flexor contraction and extensor inhibition."[11] Children learn to control their sensations and emotions through verbal and nonverbal cues. Without being told how, a child can learn to stop crying almost on command. This is possible only if there is a deep control that immobilizes the expression: the abdominals contract, the breath is suppressed, and tissue freezes. The reciprocal relationship between the diaphragm and the psoas suggest that immobilizing one will, by necessity, influence the functioning of the other. Wilhelm Reich in his book, *The Discovery of the Orgone: The Function of the Orgasm,* explains this process:

> The way in which our children accomplish this 'blocking off of sensation in the belly' by way of respiration and abdominal pressure is typical and universal....The biological function of respiration is that of introducing oxygen and of eliminating carbon dioxide from the organism. Chemically speaking, combustion is everything that consists in the formation of compounds of body substance with oxygen. In combustion, energy is created. Without oxygen, there is no combustion, and consequently no production of energy. In the organism, energy is created through the combustion of foodstuffs. In this process, heat and kinetic energy are created. Bio-electricity, also, is created in this process of combustion. If respiration is reduced, less oxygen is introduced; only as much as is needed for the maintenance of life. If a smaller amount of energy is created in the organism, the vegetative impulses are less intense and consequently easier to master.... The function of reducing the production of

energy in the organism, and thus, of reducing the production of anxiety.[12]

Because breath is an ancient function, it is strongly recommended that a person stay away from 'breathing' exercises. It is important to note that if a person does work directly with the breath he or she does so under the guidance of a qualified therapist. There is no forcible way to change the condition of the breath and most breathing exercises only interrupt a natural process increasing control to an already dysfunctional, overstimulated system.

It is essential to understand that, although sometimes appearing helpful, having a cathartic release is not the same as achieving recovery and resolution. In fact, a cathartic release can lead to a more disrupted system. A helpful strategy is to notice when a person hold his or her breath and to simply soften and let that breath go. In other words, focusing on the long exhale allows a person to begin to breathe properly. Relaxing muscular tension by softening and releasing the psoas is also a profound step toward reestablishing natural breathing.

The idea that it is just as absurd to learn to breathe as it is to learn to make a person's blood circulate is a concept shared by many somatic educators. In their book *The Body Has Its Reasons*, somatic educators Therese Bertherat and Carol Bernstein explain:

> Breathing needs not to be taught but liberated. It's imperfect because it's blocked. And it's blocked by causes that are foreign to the respiratory function. It is blocked by the shortening of the posterior muscles. The only way to treat a breathing inadequacy is, therefore, to make these muscles supple.[13]

Fear Response

For muscles to regain their suppleness they need to soften and move; the spine needs to fully bear weight and the pelvis needs to be free to respond. This allows all the diaphragmatic muscles within the pelvic floor to find their buoyant freedom. Only then can the pelvis floor and genital/anal area be experienced as open, vulnerable, and alive.

When the the genitals and adductor muscles (muscles attaching from the pubis along the inside of the femur or thigh bone) are frozen in fear, the pelvis becomes rigid and immobilized. Therefore, sensations in and around the genitals, except by direct stimulation, can no longer be experienced. In essence, sexual energy becomes blocked by the constricted psoas and frozen pelvis.

Suppression of sexual energy influences a person's whole sense of safety and well-being. A body frozen in fear will be overwhelmed by any powerful sensations. Sexual energy is a force of nature, which is both electric and dynamic; it must circulate. If sexual energy is blocked by muscular tension and cannot move freely through the pelvis, genitals, and legs, it will move upward through the body and stimulate the cardiovascular system. Reich explains this dynamic process:

> Sexuality and anxiety present two opposite directions of vegetative excitation.... The same excitation which appears in the genital as pleasure, manifests itself as anxiety if it stimulates the cardiovascular system. That is, in the latter case it appears as the exact opposite of pleasure.[14]

A healthy psoas is essential for full orgasmic potency. A full orgasm, when the whole body participates in an undulating reflex that takes over and voluntary control is given up, is only possible when the psoas is supple and the pelvis capable of undulating. Once again, the work of Feldenkrais reiterates the importance of releasing rigidity and muscular tension in the pelvis:

> By eliminating contraction and rigidity in the pelvic region, an obstacle interfering with reflex discharge of motor impulses, essential to normal orgastic release of tension in the sexual act, is removed; the way to complete maturity, sexual and otherwise, is cleared.[15]

When the psoas spontaneously releases without the use of invasive or manipulative techniques, people often report elusive feelings of fear and anxiety. In the book, *The Body Reveals,* authors Ron Kurtz and Hector Prestera MD describe this experience:

> Often trembling in the lower half of the body takes place. The pelvis may begin to jerk spasmodically or rock and the legs vibrate. This is usually accompanied by anxiety or panic at first, marked by a holding of the breath....[16]

At first, this 'excitation' flows chaotically, but then gradually transforms into sensations that flow smoothly throughout the body. The genital and anal areas can now be sensed as the pelvis relaxes and opens in both depth, width, and breadth. Feelings of vulnerability can often accompany these sensations as well as associations and attitudes concerning sexual behavior. In turn, personal discovery takes place as the capacity to sense is reestablished.

Fear Response

To reestablish personal integrity, it is necessary for a person to question where the said energetic disruptions originate and to be able to sense and therefore establish the source of the fear. By focusing on these energetic rhythms, a person balances not only sexual energy, but also his or her emotional energy.

From the point of view of Oriental Philosophy, emotions are qualities of organ meridian functioning. Their manifestations depend upon whether or not energy is lowing freely without obstruction. Thus, fear is observed as an imbalance of energy (Qi) that travels unceasingly through the meridians or pathways of the body. Author, Felix Mann, in his book *Acupuncture: The Ancient Chinese Art of Healing and How it Works Scientifically* explains that:

> The ancient Chinese made not precise distinction between arteries, veins, lymphatics, nerves, tendons or meridians. They were concerned rather with a system of forces in the body, those forces which enable a man to move, to breathe, to digest his food, to think. As in other so-called primitive systems of medicine, like the Egyptians or the Aztec, the anatomical structures which make these physiological processes possible were not described in detail. They concentrated instead on this elaborate system of forces, whose interplay regulates all the functions of the body.... Qi (life energy) is one of the fundamental concepts of Chinese thought. The manifestation of any invisible force, whether it be the growth of a plant, the movement of an arm or the deafening thunder of a storm, is called Qi.[17]

Thus fear is not simply a physical or emotional expression, it is a flow of energy that pulsates throughout the body. What a person often experiences as tension is actually blocked energy (Qi). Because of this, if a person is unaccustomed to sensing subtle flows of energy, he or she may miss out on experiencing sensation as a full embodiment of pleasure.

To perceive distinct energy flows involves reestablishing long-lost ties with sensation. This is a process that cannot be done for someone else. Although other people can assist, it is impossible to send the body in for a tune-up as if it is an automobile. For real contact to be established, the nervous system must mature. A key for reestablishing core integrity is to become aware of the present moment through sensation(s).

Many people refer to the lower parts of their body as 'down there,' revealing that such people live as though they exist from only the waistline up. This disconnect inadvertently helps people escape from the very relationship that makes it possible for them to be nourished and thrive. In fact, it is the belly core that is the center of not only sustenance, but also of movement and balance. This "right center of gravity" is experienced as a physical sensation and is perceived as an inward attitude known in Japanese as *"Hara."* Hara literally means belly and is physically centered slightly below the navel in the same area where the psoas resides. This relationship is illuminated in Karlfried Graf Von Durkheim's book, *Hara: The Vital Centre Of Man*:

> Thus we can see how people offend against the harmonious relationship between heaven and earth either by straining and stretching upwards or sagging downwards.... in both these cases the right centre of gravity-the one connecting the upper and lower is lacking. When it is present the energies pointing to heaven and those affirming the earth meet in harmony. What is

above is supported from below. What is below has a natural upward tendency. The figure grows upwards from below as the crown of a tree rises from a vertical trunk, deeply rooted. Thus the right posture expresses man's Yes to his bi-polar wholeness, his place between heaven and earth.[18]

Functional movement and a sense of balance can only occur when a person is centered in his or her Hara. The psoas sustains this profound connection. When the psoas is supple and dynamic and the pelvic basin is centered and integrated, a person's energy is said to flow harmoniously through the Hara, replacing fear with a sense of fluidity and wholeness.

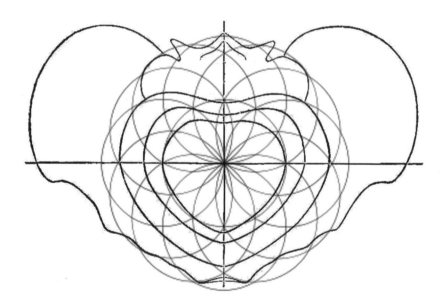

The Center Pelvic Basin

Chapter 5: Childhood Conditioning

A quintessential connection takes place while within the mother's womb: nourishment is received through the umbilical cord directly into the fetus' core. Therefore when nourishment is not forthcoming the mother's and fetus' core are directly impacted, which not only diminishes energetic vitality, but also influences the psoas muscle. Authors Ron Kurtz and Hector Prestera M.D. in their book, *The Body Reveals: An Illustrated Guide To The Psychology Of The Body,* explain this concept:

> If, in the uterus and early extrauterine environment, we were poorly nourished, we will find it emotionally difficult to receive any energies. Somewhere within us the experience of not receiving full warmth and love is imprinted. We will be untrusting, unable to open ourselves to the available nourishment around us.[19]

Whether this lack of nourishment can be attributed to the emotions a woman has toward her unborn child or to the condition of her own impoverished pelvis, the psoas influences a woman's health throughout her pregnancy, the birth, the growing fetus, and ultimately the newborn infant's health (see Chapter 7).

One of the essential influences the psoas has on both pregnancy and the fetus in utero is how the baby is carried to term. Although pregnancy offers an opportunity, due to the additional weight, to soften and lengthen the psoas naturally, this can only occur if a woman is structurally positioned so that her bones are supported and balanced. If a woman does not experience the support of her bones, she will collapse under the additional weight and her constricted psoas will thrust her belly out in front of her. This does not mean that the belly should not enlarge to accommodate the demands of the growing fetus, but that

Childhood Conditioning

when the psoas is supple, support and space comes from deep within the pelvic basin. Therefore when the psoas lengthens in response to pregnancy, the growing infant rests nestled within a woman's core.

Developmental neuro-pathways shape and expand an infant's awareness from the very beginning as a smell/touch sensory-oriented being into a smell/touch/sight sensory-oriented being. The instant the birth process begins, a baby's life is conditioned. It takes an infant nearly three years to develop voluntary control of his or her posture. The vertical standing posture develops through a progression of stages by which posture is coordinated through simple bodily reflexes until higher coordinating centers regulate voluntary movement. The impressions gained from motor behavior during the first five years of a child's life therefore, forms the basis for all future movement.

Unlike most animals whose nervous system and brain are more complete and defined at birth (a colt, for example, can stand and walk shortly after birth), human newborns are dependent upon adults for an extended period of time. For instance, walking does not take place immediately, but evolves over an extended period of developmental stages. This 'open system' provides an incredible ability to adapt to varied life experiences and to develop in unique and individual ways.

Each stage of motor development builds on the one prior to it. The fundamental and sequential stages leading to upright locomotion include: pivoting in the prone position, crawling, creeping on hands and knees, standing and balancing on two legs, standing and balancing on one leg, walking, and running. Inherent movement, which is the basic way the human body moves in space and time, is limited to only a few simple patterns that are then recombined and organized to create more sophisticated movement. At each stage, a greater development of equilibrium is required to respond to gravity. Infants begin exploring gravity as soon as their head lifts and orients ('facing') to the horizon. This is first achieved by extending the spine and head in the prone position as well as by bilaterally flexing and extending the arms and legs. By engaging the extensors muscles, infants begin to gain the muscle strength to challenge gravity.[20]

The bio-intelligent human organism intrinsically knows how to align and right itself in space and time. The nervous system is equipped to do the job and thus does not need to be taught how to move, but simply allowed to explore movement. What is consciously determined by the human being then is the direction, range, force, speed, and timing of the movement.

It is through imitation and repetition that the nervous system establishes its habits of postures, attitudes, and movements that may or may not be appropriate or even efficient for a given situation. Moshe Feldenkrais in his book, *Body and Mature Behavior,* explains:

> In most of the acts taught to us, the insistence is on a procedure similar to that which the adult considers to be satisfactory. The child is urged in one way or another to do something to itself, and become master of its vegetative system- often before he has even the rudiments of control of his of voluntary muscles. Some parents will pay more attention to this or that activity, some to another, depending on the age, the society and the knowledge prevailing at the time. It is thus a matter of pure chance, with a large bias towards the imitation of the adults concerned, as to which particular pattern of doing the child will strive for,

even in the best cases. It is most likely that he will adopt a particular manner of doing in order to satisfy or imitate some adult. Repetition, however, soon facilitates the flow of nervous impulses, as if the associated paths straighten, deepen and become preferred.[21]

Each stage of development is a preparation and a foundation for the next stage. Crawling, for example, is the stage that matures the ball and socket hip joint proprioception. It is through the process of crawling that the nervous system and motor skills develop. Therefore a playpen or any confining apparatus ultimately limits crawling and thus proprioceptive development. The hip sockets become fully mobile and sufficiently extended only when there is an adequate period of crawling.

When babies are not free to move spontaneously, but are restrained in apparatus that define or curtail movement (such as day containers, carseats, and portable beds) for long periods of time, motor skill development can become compromised. Additionally, babies who are not placed on their stomachs cannot explore belly-to-head extension, which enables them to naturally arch through the spine, lengthening their psoas.

Many children are encouraged to sit up and walk prematurely before the action is initiated and carried out unaided. Doing so can be the first step to misusing the psoas muscle. Although a young child may initially recruit the psoas in an effort to stabilize his or her growing bones, a child inherently lets go of the the psoas as the bones become weight-bearing. However, this can only occur if a child's nervous systems has the opportunity to naturally mature. For example, when a baby's hands are held above his or her head (with the arms above the shoulders) and 'walked,' it does not quicken the baby's developmental process, but actually interrupts fundamental maturation. Prolonged standing before the bones are weight-bearing also conditions a baby's neuro-muscular patterns. Premature standing (when the lumbar curve of the spine has not yet formed and the muscles of the lower abdominal wall have yet to develop) conditions a toddler to become muscularly dependent upon large external leg muscles and his or her psoas. If instead, a toddler spontaneously stands and walks (approximately 12 to 18 months) it is with a sense of balance, agility, and confidence. When a toddler falls, he or she will be more likely to sit straight down rather than collapse. When a level of developmental proprioception is achieved, it will reveal itself in all facets of life: motor skills, psychological maturity, and cognitive development.

Walking is primarily an act of falling and catching: at the moment when the body begins to fall forward, the neutral psoas softens and the righting reflexes fire; the vestibular system coordinates the catching phase as muscles activate and the system rights itself in space. Thus human movement emerges from a dynamic core rather than being pushed and pulled along by the legs and arms.

Midline Axis

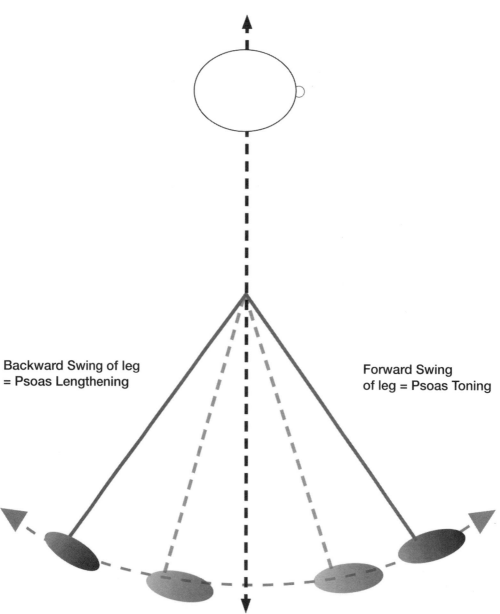

Backward Swing of leg
= Psoas Lengthening

Forward Swing
of leg = Psoas Toning

Released (Neutral) Psoas moving as a Pendulum

Chapter 6: Releasing The Psoas

A short, dry, or constricted psoas muscle can become, once again, supple and responsive. The first step before attempting any type of psoas stretch, however, is to soften the tissue. The Constructive Rest Position (CRP) coined by somatic educator, Lulu Sweigard, is a spontaneous position that uses gravity to release extraneous muscle tension, which in turn supports a neutral spine.

PREPARATION: Choose a place to be in CRP that is quiet and safe. Fold a blanket the full length of the body from head to tail. Be sure to always have padding when resting on a hard floor and to take shoes off.

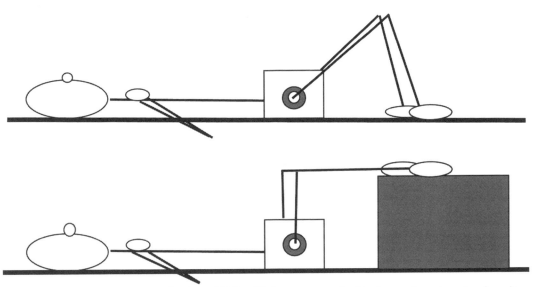

Option: CRP with legs supported helps reduce low back pain

Begin in CRP: Lie down on a padded floor with the knees bent at a 45 degree angle and both feet on the floor. Separate the feet and knees the width of the hip sockets (located on the front of the pelvis). If needed, place a towel no thicker than 1 1/2 inches under the back of the head. Neatly fold the towel, so that it is flat and place it under the upper half of the skull rather than under the neck. The function of the towel is to support the cervical spine so that the head and pelvis are level and parallel with the floor. The head should be is neutral and should not tilt forward toward the chest (using towel) or backward toward the floor (without using towel). Only use a towel if needed. Allow the arms to rest at the sides of the body, on top of the hip sockets, or resting over the chest. Allow the eyes to remain soft but open. Rest for 10-20 minutes. When ready to leave the position, roll to one side and rest for 1-3 minutes before getting up slowly. Do not pull up out of the position. Instead, push down on the floor with the upper hand to get out of the position. Once standing, take time to observe the changes in skeletal alignment. If prone to back pain, walk on a flat surface for 5-10 minutes and avoid a fast, deep flexing movements.

As the psoas releases superfluous energy, the sensations experienced may cause feelings of vulnerability. If physical aches or emotional feelings arise from the conditioned muscular patterns in CRP, become quiet and simply follow the sensations throughout the body. Notice the stream of images, thoughts, and emotions that move through the body as the awareness of sensation increases.

There is no need to change anything or to be absorbed by these associations. Instead, keep returning to the qualities of sensation coming from within body as well as sensations from outside the body, such as air currents, the warmth of sunlight, odors, and sounds. Match the external impressions with the quality of sensations and feelings inside. Ideally, a balance will begin to occur between what is experienced internally and what is being received from external stimuli. By balancing the intensity of the internal world with the sensory impressions from the external world, there will be a moment where the two interface: this is the process of awakening. Being in the moment forges new nerve pathways and frees old conditioning to dissolve.

BEST TIME: The best times to rest in CRP is during the day, just before an activity, such as yoga or pilates, and after the day's work (just before dinner). Do not spend time in CRP just before going to sleep as doing so can disrupt sleep by awakening and energizing the system.

BENEFITS: CRP relieves psoas tension, creates core neutrality, and reestablishes skeletal balance. Spending time in CRP every day revitalizes and prepares a person for the day's activities and/or provides recovery time from stimulation and stress. Lying on the floor frees the central nervous system from stimuli that evokes habitual response patterns to gravity so that subtle sensations can be experienced. CRP may be used before teaching or working with clients and students as a subtle, non-invasive method of assisting a person in releasing his or her own psoas.

KEY: Use no force. If the back naturally arches, do not attempt to force the spine to the floor. Begin developing proprioceptive awareness by noticing the sensation of weight. Allow thoughts to quiet and bring awareness to resting on the floor. CRP is a 'being' position, there is nothing to do. Overtime as the psoas releases the spine will release as well and lengthen along the floor. Force is neither needed nor helpful.

Releasing The Psoas

Begin in CRP to awaken the hip sockets and articulate movement of the leg from the core. With the pelvis centered, extend one leg at a time, sliding the foot along the floor. Place awareness and soften at the front of the hip sockets. Use a soften-move-pause rhythm, noticing when the leg moves freely without the pelvis.

Tips for Exploring the Psoas in CRP

- Begin with a neutral spine in Constructive Rest Position.

- Notice weight: what senses weighted - what senses suspended?

- Bring awareness to the lower psoas by resting fingers gently on the hip sockets.

- Soften the eyes: do not stare at the ceiling or wear glasses.

- As the psoas releases and frees the hip sockets, notice how weight begins to pass through the legs grounding the feet.

- Match sensations, feelings, and thoughts with incoming sensory impressions from light, sound, touch, taste, and smell.

KEY: When done properly, there is no pulling in the low back. If the back arcs, begin again putting more awareness toward softening the psoas as it passes over the front of the hip socket. Releasing the psoas allows the leg to move separately from pelvis. The purpose of the exploration is not to extend the leg fully or to hold the pelvis from moving, but to mature the hip socket by learning to voluntarily soften the psoas.

RELEASING THE LOWER PSOAS:

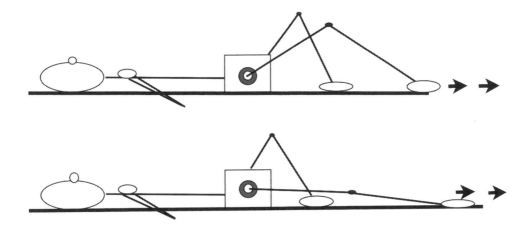

DO: Extend the leg only moving the leg at the hip sockets. Pause, soften, and bring awareness to the front of the hip socket.

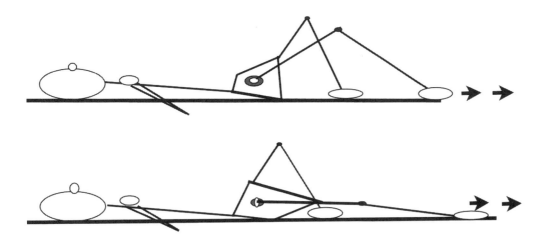

DO NOT: Keep extending the leg if the pelvis moves. STOP - extend the leg only as far as it will go without involving the pelvis.

Releasing The Psoas

SOFTENING THE PSOAS:

Begin in CRP. Softening a dry, constricted psoas is a process that begins with movement. A soft, inflated (no more than 1/4th), 7-10 inch inflatable exercise ball, such as the Slo-mo™ brand works effectively for creating fluid movement along the spine. Place the softly inflated ball under the upper psoas (right behind the solar plexus) and let the weight of the lower ribs rest on the ball. By giving up the weight, it is easy to gently rock from side to side. Let the rocking become a wave-like motion. Use a soft 'haw' sound on the exhale breath. Explore the area for 2-5 minutes and then move the ball down along the spine - stopping along the way to rest and then repeat the wave-like motion until the ball is placed under the pelvis. With legs on the floor or up on a support, let the weight rest on the ball, and rock in a wave-like undulating movement.

KEY: The ball should not feel imposing: reduce the air in the ball until the spine can rest comfortably.

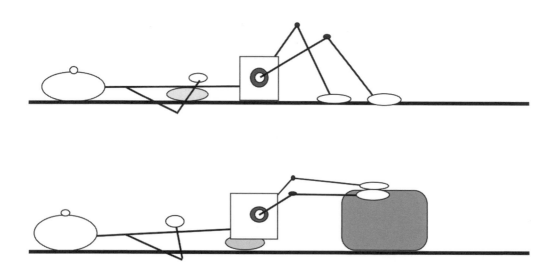

RELEASING THE UPPER PSOAS:

Begin in CRP focusing awareness on the solar plexus. Lift the arms straight up, (the distance apart of the shoulder sockets) with the palms facing each other. Sense the weight of each arm as it releases at the shoulder socket. Move both arms over the head toward the floor. Allow the weight of the arms to soften the solar plexus and upper psoas. Do not push the arms to the floor by arching the low back. Keep the spine neutral while softening the solar plexus and let go of any superfluous muscular tension. To return the arms to the start position, keep the weight centered within the pelvis and the feet. Lightly push the feet into the ground to lift the arms, maintaining a soft, supple psoas.

KEY: The eyes and head follow the movement of the arms. The psoas releases through the pelvis toward the feet even though the arms move up over the head, awakening sexual energy in the genitals and pelvis floor.

DO: Open the throat, letting the eyes follow the fingers.

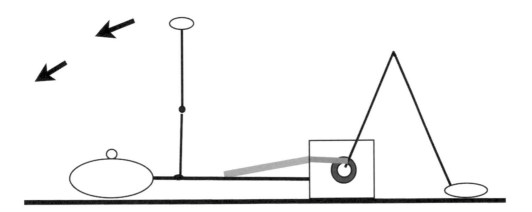

Releasing The Psoas

TONING THE PSOAS:

Begin in CRP softening and releasing the psoas. When the leg can fully extend without involving the pelvis, release at the hip socket and lift the extended leg the height of that hip socket. The neutral psoas should free the leg to lift up and down, side to side, and diagonally. Simultaneously sense the weight on the side with the bent leg and foot. Switch sides.

KEY: The pelvis should stay centered and the spine neutral when the psoas falls back along the spine as the leg lifts off the floor.

DO: Maximize awareness of the psoas by lifting leg no higher than 3-5 inches

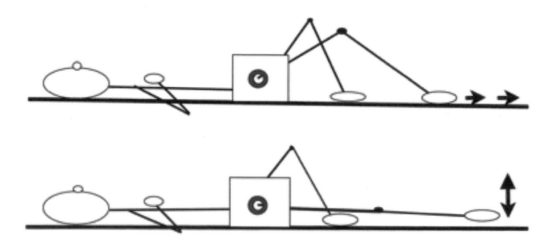

DO NOT: Tone if pelvis tilts or torques. Keep the pelvis balanced.

Releasing The Psoas

RELEASING AND TONING THE PSOAS:

Begin in CRP softening and releasing the psoas. Roll over onto the hands and knees, distribute the weight evenly through all four contact points. Soften through the ball and socket hip joint and release the psoas and lengthen one leg. The pelvis should stay balanced and the spine neutral. Provide abdominal tone to maintain a neutral spine. Return leg and switch sides. Once lengthening is achieved, move the extended leg up and down (maximum of 3-5 inches) and side to side keeping a released, supple psoas. Switch sides.

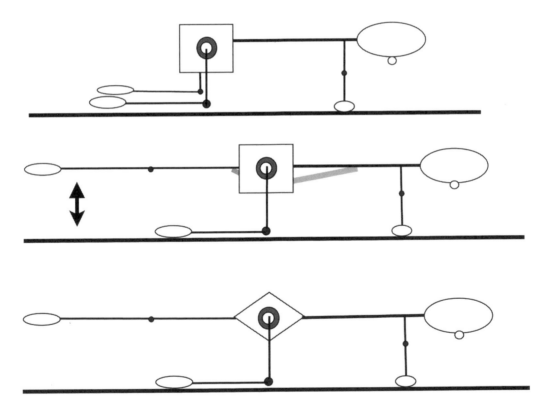

DO NOT: Continue if pelvis tilts, dips, or torques.

LENGTHENING THE PSOAS:

Begin by softening and releasing in CRP to create suppleness in the tissue and responsiveness in the spine. Explore releasing the lower and upper psoas in CRP. Leg lengthening frees the bones to align in a weight-bearing position. The aligned joints are then free to move without compensation. Lengthening the whole psoas articulates the leg from the trunk, relaxes the abdominal core, expands the rib cage, and increases range of motion.

Place a tightly rolled yoga mat directly under the pelvis (use 1 or 2 mats rolled as one - depending upon height and width needed). Allow the pelvis to drop over the front edge of the mat. Doing so, opens the front of the hip socket and lengthens the lower psoas.

Lengthen the upper psoas (on the same side) by extending the arm over the head (see upper psoas release exploration). Maintain CRP on the opposite side. Open the throat (to do so look up with the eyes toward the extended hand) and relax the jaw.

Starting from the breastbone or heart area, begin a gentle spiral toward the extended side - Looking up at the elbow.

KEY: Keep awareness in the front of the hip sockets. Never strain or tense the lower back. The pelvis must be stable and the trunk unified. A unified trunk frees the psoas providing integrity to the whole muscle.

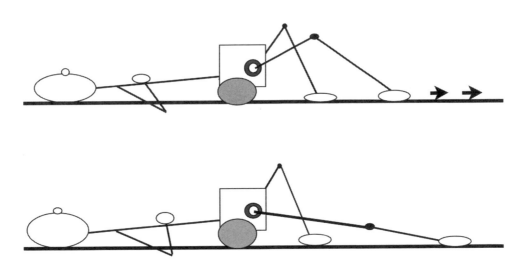

DO: Release the lower psoas at the hip socket by extending one leg.

DO: Release the upper psoas by extending one arm.

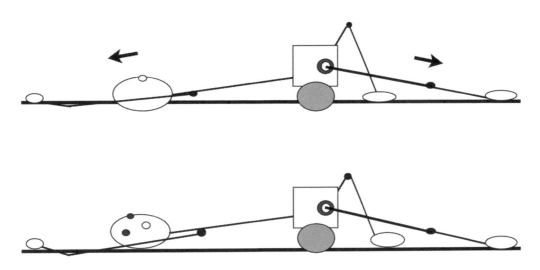

DO NOT: Pull or lock the joints - keep joints soft.

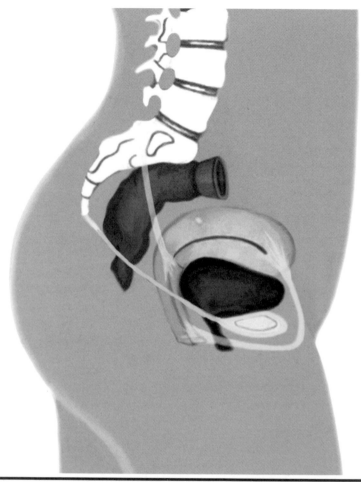

Female Organs - with permission
Artists, Nikelle Gessner and Christine Kent (author of *Saving The Whole Woman),* are a mother-daughter team that has worked to draw the accurate female pelvis for over ten years. Kent discovered that anatomy charts and surgical procedures are often based upon an inaccurate perspective of the female pelvis and the positioning of the female organs, which sit forward tucked under the pubis.
More information can be found Whole Woman®

Chapter 7: Reproductive Health

MENSTRUATION: Softening and releasing the psoas can successfully relieve menstrual cramps. Women who have previously taken drugs for severe cramps have found that releasing their psoas helps them to be pain and drug free. As part of the fear response, the psoas reflects fears associated with menstruation, reproduction, and sexuality. It is often a constricted psoas, not the uterus itself, that presses on the reproductive organs impeding blood circulation and irritating the nerves.

Becoming 'she who bleeds but does not die' requires that a young girl let go of her childhood innocence and emerge into the world as a fertile woman. Beginning her menstrual cycle between the young age of 9 and 16, a girl may feel insecurity, shame, and embarrassment associated with bleeding. The feeling of being out of control can be frightening. What may already feel like an overwhelming experience, can be compounded by religious and sexual taboos. Additionally, most cultures do not have rituals that acknowledge and celebrate this profound change in a young woman's life. Because the psoas reflects the fear response, working with the psoas may actually be a direct way for a woman to access her true feelings regarding menstruation.

PREGNANCY: Due to the additional weight in the pelvis, a pregnant woman's attention naturally goes into the belly offering an opportunity to spontaneously lengthen the psoas. By increasing her awareness of the center of gravity, a pregnant woman can begin to expand and deepen her sense of self and her innate power.

Reproductive Health

Pregnancy is a time for growth, letting go, and starting new. Because the weight of pregnancy helps free the psoas, it can be a time to stimulate and deepen an inner sense of self. Thus working with the psoas offers a woman and her baby a rich environment that is both spacious, and nourishing.

Once the belly grows, adjusting the constructive rest position becomes necessary. The use of a chair helps support the legs early on, and resting in a partially reclined position, supported by a large wedge or pillows, can help when it is no longer possible or safe to rest fully reclined it is important for the spine to be supported evenly from head to coccyx.

KEY: As the pregnancy progresses, a woman needs to reduce the time spent in the position from up to twenty minutes a session to five or ten minutes at a time.

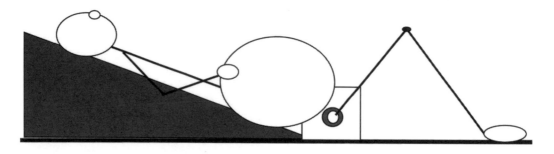

During Pregnancy: Use Wedge for reclining in CRP

FIRST TRIMESTER: When a pregnant woman's psoas is constricted it reduces the internal space available for the organs, viscera, and the womb with its growing fetus. By softening and releasing the psoas, a woman can not only benefit from the internal space gained, but also can ease nausea as well as improve digestion and sleep.

SECOND TRIMESTER: A supple psoas provides more internal space for the growing fetus, helps to stimulate organ functioning, and allows the spine the freedom to shift and create more support throughout the core. Moreover, releasing and tonifying the psoas relieves minor aches that contribute to a sense of overall well-being.

THIRD TRIMESTER: Maintaining a supple psoas helps to relieve pressure from the discomfort of an ever-growing belly and increases overall energy. Keeping the psoas healthy gives the hip sockets the freedom to move and transfer weight into the legs, helping to relieve leg and back pains. Supporting the release of the psoas also helps to stimulate intuitive awareness and primal knowing.

Focusing on the psoas can help a woman prepare for birth. The psoas muscle guides the baby as it spins down into the birth canal. By releasing fears and pent up emotions, a woman attunes herself to the energy of labor (the power from within that aids a woman through transition), which helps calm and center her in preparation for childbirth.

LABOR AND BIRTH: Learning to release the psoas muscle enhances a woman's birth experience, shortens labor, and, in many cases, can be an alternative to chemically intrusive methods of induction. It should certainly be the first step before an induction is considered. A released iliopsoas assists the pelvic bones in opening, facilitating the baby's movement down through the birth canal.

Choosing a birth location is often a fear-based decision rather than a choice guided by instinct. When a woman makes a decision based on her intuitive gut feelings, her choice can empower and strengthen her for the journey of birth into motherhood.

BREASTFEEDING: Although there is no obvious connection between the psoas and breastfeeding, a supple psoas ultimately enhances the breastfeeding experience. Similar to giving birth, listening to intuition is a vital mothering tool that helps a woman respond appropriately to her newborn regardless of current trends, taboos, religious, or cultural beliefs. Rather than following the whim of a culture, tapping into her primal roots helps a woman listen to her own instinctive wisdom. The more centered a new mother is, the less likely her own doubts and other people's opinions will stop her milk from flowing. Since nothing short of breast surgery prevents a woman from breastfeeding, success is essentially an issue of a woman feeling emotionally secure in herself and supported by loved ones. Even though at times it can feel like a 'lost art,' the body instinctively knows how to breastfeed. Breastfeeding is a gift of nourishment and love that relaxes the baby's as well as the mother's psoas. Moreover, it fosters a deep-felt satisfaction that bonds baby and mother.

MENOPAUSE: During a great time of change, menopause, demands that a woman pay attention to all aspects of her life. As the psoas is central to living in the core, it may be called upon during this time of metamorphous. The organs and glands, especially the kidneys and adrenals, adjusting to their new rhythms, send messages to the brain via nerve impulses. In response, the vertebrae may torque (via the psoas). Thus a dance takes place that can either enhance a woman's sense of self or create feelings of instability and chaos. Releasing old fears calms the nervous system preparing it for the 'change of life.' Working with the psoas can support a woman in feeling centered and grounded with her transformed body.

PROSTATE HEALTH: Groin pain and other symptoms of prostate dysfunction may be improved by working with the iliopsoas complex. Due to its close proximity to the ureter, colon, spermatic cord, and related nerves, the iliopsoas influences every aspect of male sexual and urinary health. Prolonged and dysfunctional sitting disrupts reproductive health, compressing organs and viscera. Resting weight on the sacrum, tucking the tailbone, collapsing the spine, and tightening the hip sockets are all characteristics of dysfunctional sitting that disrupt reproductive health. Similar to women, men must also keep their pelvic floor healthy by sitting on top and in front of the sits bone: hip sockets extended, psoas released, and the pelvic basin balanced (for example, not sitting with a wallet in the back pocket). Letting the tailbone float and the iliacus muscle fan open helps to maximize the length and the breadth of the pelvic basin. Thus providing the organs with proper placement and good circulation.

Note: Groin pain can also be caused by abbesses located in the actual psoas tissue.

Reproductive Health

AGING: Staying weight-bearing is essential for reproductive health and is vital for both female and male skeletal health regardless of age. 65% of adults lose the movement in their hip sockets resulting in hip replacement, and many are diagnosed with osteoporosis. Keeping the psoas supple, keeps the hips functionally engaged and the spine dynamically weight-bearing. Therefore increasing skeletal, visceral, and hormonal health.

The rocking chair is a great tool for releasing the psoas not only for the pregnant woman or breastfeeding mother, but also for the elderly man or woman. Any person with limited movement and/or a dry, constricted psoas will benefit from rocking. To keep the psoas soft, supple, and responsive, use a simple wood rocker to produce a rhythmic wave-like motion.

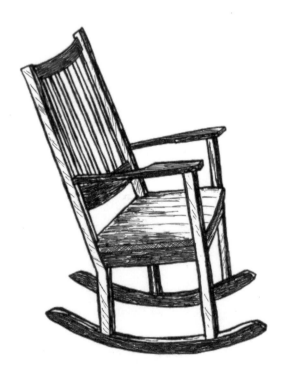

Chapter 8: Application

CHAIRS: Many chairs are designed for stacking rather than sitting. When selecting a chair, first note the bottom of the seat. Avoid bucket seats and any seats that form a curved bottom. Bucket shaped seats collapse the pelvis, narrowing the iliacus and encourages a person to sit on his or her sacrum rather than the tuberosities (sit bones).

The seat of a chair needs to offer a solid base of support for the sit bones and be at the correct height for the feet to be in contact with the floor. Only when the pelvis is balanced can the psoas stay released and supple. Therefore, sitting on top and in front of the sit bones, with the hip sockets slightly higher than the knees, maintains a centered pelvis.

When the feet do not touch the floor, a sense of rebound is lost throughout the skeletal system. For example, employing a kneeling stool as an office chair not only does not allow the feet to be grounded, but also stresses the knees over time. Ball chairs, when used over long periods of time, can also disrupt proprioception and skeletal health. An office chair needs to offer support and proprioceptively inform the spine in space and time. A favorite psoas-savvy desk stool is the Swopper.®

To maintain a healthy psoas when driving a car, fill the bucket seat with a firm wedge and position the front of the seat slightly down, which will help to keep the hip sockets open. Leaning back while driving engages and thus misuses the psoas. For responsive driving, keep the psoas neutral by tilting the back of the seat slightly forward to free the psoas, so it can stay released.

Note: Use a firm wedge to modify the seat and/or height of a chair

Application

DESKS: When sitting at a desk, gaining upper psoas support begins with a balanced pelvis. The head and trunk of the body must be in relationship to one another, so the spine is supported and the upper psoas is released. Keeping the eyes neutral, by modifying the height of a desk, can help to avoid overriding neck-head reflexes. For example, lifting a computer screen to a height that encourages the head/trunk to remain upright and balanced protects the eyes and neck from becoming strained.

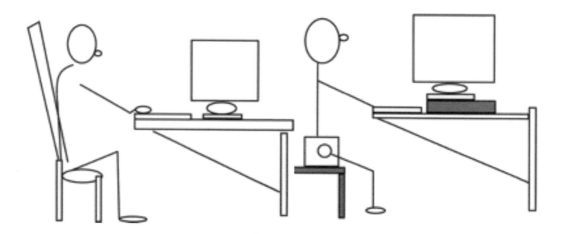

TRIKES & BIKES: Children love to ride bicycle-like toys as early as they begin to walk. Because of this, it is key to choose a trike or push-car that allows the child to sit firmly on his or her pelvis and that is moved by the feet. As the child grows, the trike or bike seat needs to be readjusted to a height that keeps the pelvis balanced, the hips open, the hip sockets slightly higher than the knees. The leg muscles should fully extend. Moreover, adjusting the handlebars allow the arms to come straight from the shoulder, which supports the upper body. The same idea holds true for adults as well as cyclists.

Application

SHOES: Shoes play an important role for maintaining a healthy psoas and for "pendulum" walking. Mobility in the foot is necessary for the dynamic diaphragm (arch) to be buoyant and for the sensitive nerves, located in the heel and ball of the foot, to fire properly. Stiff-soled shoes restrain the foot from rolling, pointed toed shoes restrict the toes from spreading, high heels forward-thrust the pelvis by tipping a person's center of gravity forward, and heavy and/or stiff high topped shoes can stop the ankle from bending, limiting movement not only throughout the foot, but also all the way up into the hip socket. Shoes influence the quality of movement throughout the entire leg. Because of this, the shoes a person wears can result in a lack of rhythm while walking, which disrupts and engages the psoas as well as other muscles rather than allowing free swing of the leg and foot.

The way a person walks begins when they are a toddler. A toddler's growing foot requires the freedom to roll and move. Many children's shoes do not bend or flex. A child's shoe needs to be comfortably wide, light, and able to bend in half so that proprioception through skeletal coherency, can develop mature movement, and of developmental patterns.

The everyday shoe for an adult also needs to bend in half, provide room for the toes to move, and have a neutral to slightly positive heel. Moreover, the bottom of a shoe should not be designed in such a way that it demands the foot to conform to a particular shape or movement. This may be an appropriate shoe for a specific activity such as golf, basketball, running track, or hiking but it is not appropriate for the every day walking shoe. A psoas-savvy shoe is very basic: it protects the foot from heat, cold, and rough surfaces.

CRUTCHES: One of the quickest ways that a person can lose a supple psoas is by using a cane or walker because of an injury. When a tool is required for extra support while walking, using a walking staff (or two if need be) rather than a cane or walker helps keep the psoas fully lengthened and prevents it from drying out, shrinking and constricting.

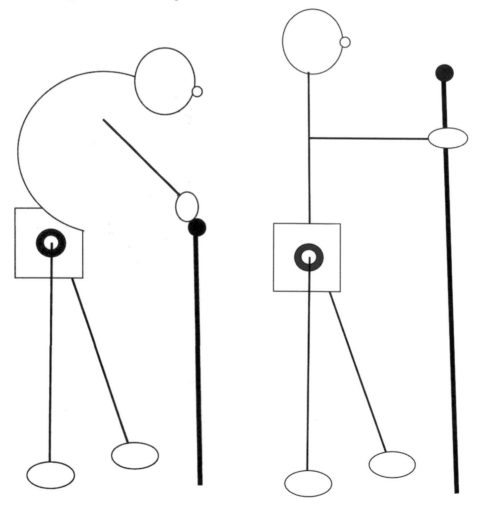

Do Not use a cane   Do Use a Walking Staff

Chapter 9: Approaches

What matters most when working with the psoas is not what a person does, but how a person does it. There are numerous types of movement and/or exercise systems as well as various methods of bodywork that can each be evaluated from the point of view of how they interact with the psoas. The reason a person chooses an activity rather than another involves his or her location, availability, personal conditioning, interests, understanding, and goals; however, what is truly important when it comes to the psoas is whether there is subtle variety and stimuli for developing and maturing sensory perception.

Solely practicing a movement does not necessarily develop awareness, create health, and sustain or increase function. In fact, repetitive movement can simply promote a faulty way of moving. Essentially, without increased awareness, repetition produces nothing new proprioceptively and can actually result in negative stress and injury. To truly discover the core from within demands that a person always begins with core awareness. The result being a supple, responsive psoas and a neutral core.

Every person needs spontaneous play, variety, and activities that provide proprioceptive enrichment. Engaging the right muscle group for a particular activity is also vital. If a person's proprioception is disrupted performing a task too difficult, he or she will "substitute" in an attempt to perform the activity. Because of this, the body will compensate by using alternative muscles. For example, when the bones are not weight-bearing, a constricted psoas and a lack of core integrity can activate the adductors (the muscles of the inner thigh) rather than engage the outward rotators (the opposing muscles to the iliacus within the hip), resulting in distortions and restrictions throughout the pelvis, leg, hip socket, and pubis. An illustration of the inappropriate use of the adductors appears when a person cannot experience the legs as weight-bearing while in CRP. To stop substituting muscles so that new motor pathways can be forged, a person has to increase proprioception, improve skeletal awareness, and soften constricted muscles.

Note: The outcome of receiving any form of work or training is only as good as the practitioner or teacher. The following descriptions are solely meant to be a guide to the psoas muscle. Please remember that feeling safe is essential and ultimately awareness is a personal process for which another person can only be of assistance.

BODYWORK (Structural & Somatic): There are many varied and popular theories for correcting the alignment of the body. Each theory encapsulates ideas that impact the psoas muscle. Although bodywork and massage techniques that work to slowly release the hip socket can be advantageous, it is also necessary to take caution. Problems can arise from attempting to palpate or trigger-point the psoas. Bruising of delicate tissue, breaking of arteries, and intestinal hernias are all associated with manipulating the psoas. Supple and juicy, only the lower section of the psoas (around the hip sockets) has extensive facia. It is a lean tissue: the tenderloin or filet mignon. Releasing the psoas using non-manipulative and non-invasive techniques are more effective, empowering, and long lasting because working with the psoas depends upon how responsive a person is to new impressions and how quickly these new impressions can be integrated. Strong, deep, and powerful work can be too overwhelming to a person and will simply be rejected by the nervous system. Thus subtle, indirect approaches are actually more beneficial because they can be assimilated and allow for integration to occur at a pace that is responsive to a person and the context of his or her life.

Approaches

- **Alexander Technique:** Frederick Matthias Alexander worked with the idea that the "Primary Control" of posture is located within the head and neck relationship. Working to release the head and neck therefore allows the spine to realign. This is a good idea and an accurate one; however, because people tend to reside in their heads, it is not necessarily the best place to start to create a sensory based change. Although the psoas is not the major focus, there is a great deal to be learned from engaging the righting reflexes.

- **Aston-Patterning:** Developed by Judith Aston, Aston-Patterning transpired out of a relationship with Ida Rolf. With a background in both dance and movement, Judith Aston's method offers a three-dimensional approach to the body in motion. Aston-Patterning approaches a person's holding patterns as a process that needs to be unraveled. Rather than focus on simple linear relationships, Aston-Patterning emphasizes full diagonal (spiral) relationships. Since the psoas is an integral part of unraveling, Aston-Patterning releases the psoas, returning it to its rightful place as a unifying factor in posture and movement. An example of Aston's perspective concerning the body, which directly influences the psoas, is that she perceives the pelvis to be in dynamic motion. In an interview with Somatic Magazine/Journal, Aston explicates:

> When the angle of the pelvic crest is parallel to the ground (horizontal) the weight is placed on the heel - this is the model for Rolfing as well as for Sweigard and Alexander. What needs to happen is a resilient positioning of the pelvis onto the the top of the legs; this would allow the chest to occupy more of it's depth, and the elbows, arms and head to realize a different freedom of movement. The weight could then go over the whole foot in a light manner. In this way, during motion, the

shock absorbers of the body would accept the impact of weight allowing the body to actually massage itself while moving.[22]

- **Energy Work:** Having a direct ability to successfully release the psoas, energy work should not be underestimated. Unlike trigger-pointing or palpating the abdomen or manipulating the psoas, energy work releases the psoas without ever touching the body. Subtle but very effective, energy work is not invasive and therefore does not elicit a person's instinctive fear response or activate his or her psoas.

- **Feldenkrais:** Working to develop awareness of the whole person, the Moshe Feldenkrais method focuses on maturing the nervous system by refining awareness. Feldenkrais considers the psoas to have a vital influence on the lumbar vertebrae by allowing the pelvis to fully extend. When the pelvis is fully extended, it creates a sense of stability in the pelvic basin, which manifests a support for the spinal vertebrae. The Feldenkrais method specifically emphasizes diagonal and lateral relationships and cross-patterning movement that increases proprioception essential for maintaining a supple psoas.

- **Lulu Sweigard:** One of the leading educators in the 1930's, Lulu Sweigard's work revolves around the "Human Movement Potential." She and her student, Mabel Todd, originally coined the term Constructive Rest Position (CRP). Sweigard and Todd both emphasize the importance of the released psoas and its ability to establish core integrity. To develop awareness, Sweigard and Todd employ imagery as a means for correcting old patterns and habits of moving, which improves the alignment of a person's posture. Although the use of imagery can be inspirational, employing imagery is fundamentally a mental process rather than a kinesthetic process and therefore is a step away from experiencing direct sensation.

- **Massage:** Numerous forms of massage can offer relaxation, a healing touch, and increase awareness. However, it is focal not to have anyone palpate and/ or manipulate the psoas muscle because to do so triggers the sympathetic nervous system (fight-flight-freeze response).

- **Ortho-Bionomy:** Borne from an Osteopathic model of working with the body, the system of Ortho-Bionomy was developed by Arthur Lincoln Pauls. Working to restore natural balance through unraveling and stimulating the self-correcting reflexes, Ortho-Bionomy offers a very psoas-savvy approach for reestablishing core integrity.

- **Somatics**: Coining the word "somatics," derived from the Greek word "soma" that translates as "living body," Thomas Hanna developed a system for becoming self aware through making small movements by way of the voluntary motor system. Hanna Somatics offers a self-help approach for developing kinesthetic awareness, which is pivotal for a healthy psoas.

- **Structural Integration (Rolfing):** This technique was developed by Dr. Ida Rolf who popularized and acknowledged the psoas muscle as the foundation for structural integrity. Rolf's ideas of posture are built around engaging the psoas 'properly.' For many people the word psoas is synonymous with Rolfing. Rolfing has radically changed over the years and has branched into the study of fascia and connective tissue. However, regardless of the style utilized, Rolfing tends to be a 'fix-it' model by which the practitioner activates the psoas through direct manipulation. Directly attempting to manipulate the psoas, however, contradicts the very essence of the psoas as a messenger for integrity. Because the psoas muscle is a part of the fear reflex system and the sympathetic neuro-core (the connective tissue enclosing the spinal cord, psoas, and kidneys) when a practitioner directly palpates the tissue, this sabotages the instinctive response of the psoas. Rather than utilizing invasive techniques, empowering a person to sense the capacity to release his or her own psoas enhances core integrity and results in resolution of the fear response.

CONTINUUM MOVEMENT: A movement pioneer, Emilie Conrad is the founder of "Continuum," which is the study of fluid movement. The bases of her work is to hydrate all connective tissue and to shift the perception of body as object to body as self-referential: a living process. Continuum is an excellent way to free the spine and psoas, breathe the bones into health, and nourish the parasympathetic nervous system.

CYCLING: Long distance cycling is a quadricep-dominant activity. Unless the bones are in proper alignment and the bike is sized and adjusted to fit properly, cycling can overdevelop leg muscles. Overdeveloped flexor muscles pull the pelvis forward and the knee joint into inward rotation, torquing the leg bones and putting pressure on the knees. Creating balance for a muscle dominant activity, such as cycling, entails extending the flexor muscles (full hip extension), so the leg has the opportunity to move through its full range of motion rather than only contract. Developing awareness is key to being able to sense which muscles are being engaged during any movement. Muscle density, pelvic positioning, and upper body alignment will all dictate whether or not the psoas can remain supple while cycling.

Approaches

DANCE: When muscle control is used as a means for securing posture, the result is increased muscle fatigue, loss of flexibility, and inefficiency. Despite this, a popular approach to dance is to gain strong muscle control. If dancers speak of the psoas muscle at all, it is usually referred to as a muscle that requires strengthening. By contracting the upper psoas, a dancer stabilizes his or her trunk while the legs move. This is particularly true regarding ballet and related Western forms of dance in which the psoas is intentionally engaged to support weight and gain range of motion. In his article "East-West Dance Forms," Bob Cooley explains that *"In ballet, muscular contraction of the abdominal and gluteus maximus is intentional while work on the thigh is attempted. This is done to counteract the short resting length of the flexors and especially the iliopsoas muscles."*[23] To truly 'strengthen' the psoas entails gaining resiliency. Releasing, neutralizing, and lengthening core tissue allows bones to be fully weight-bearing. Strong muscles are not the same as overdeveloped muscles. One result of overdeveloped muscles is a pelvis that is controlled by dominant leg patterns. A dominant leg pattern begins at the top of the pelvis rather than at the hip sockets and thus articulation between the pelvis and the leg is lost.

- **Hawkins Technique:** One innovative approach to dance is The Hawkins Technique developed by the late Eric Hawkins. This technique focuses on working with rather than against the psoas muscle by learning to 'track' or move at the hip socket.

- **Contact Improvisation:** Another innovative approach to dance that works with weight transference to increase a sense of flow between bones and gravity is called "Contact Improvisation." To bear weight properly and fluidly, it is essential to maintain a supple psoas. Although the psoas is not spoken of directly, Contact Improvisation acknowledges the necessity for having a balanced, weight-bearing skeleton and a responsive core.

EXERCISE & SPORTS: Exercises and various sport activities emphasize strength, endurance, and speed. Additionally, the development of muscle control often takes precedence rather than skeletal balance. Gaining speed at the expense of mounting tension is often the goal. Although it is possible to work with a neutral, supple psoas, a person must first slow down until he or she can follow the quality of movement with sensory awareness. For example, when a person is playing tennis, golf, or baseball, he or she needs to be able to sense whether rotation is taking place at the ball and socket hip joint or if the movement is initiated by twisting the spine and knees. By maturing kinesthetic awareness, a person is able improve the articulation of movement patterns. By becoming aware of a person's patterns, he or she can gain new neuro-pathways. With this increased awareness is borne efficiency and speed.

MOVEMENT & MARTIAL ARTS: Jujitsu, Aikido, Qi Gong, and Tai Chi are just a few of the Eastern forms of movement that can lead to a richer and more supple expression of the psoas. Focusing on moving with the flow of gravity, these forms of movement develop awareness of the core and explore the harnessing of life energy (Qi). Although the psoas is not specifically emphasized, centering and moving from within the belly is, and thus awakens core awareness and resiliency.

PILATES: Developed by the late Joseph Pilates, the Pilates method focuses on core strength as the foundation for a healthy body. The method, originally referred to as "contrology," focuses on the quality (rather than quantity) of movement by engaging a person's attention, breath and precision. Although Pilates takes the psoas muscle into consideration, whether or not the psoas is engaged for support and control or released for neutral and supple expression depends upon the approach of the instructor.

RUNNING & WALKING: Similar to other activities, running does not in and of itself necessarily improve posture that is already poor or constricted. In fact, it often exaggerates problems due to muscle substitution. If the psoas is already constricted and dry, it will still be so during and after running. Moreover, repetitive and inappropriate development of the musculature leads to diminished sensitivity. Stress occurs in the knees, feet, and low back and thus precludes healthy functioning of the psoas. Of course, it is possible to engage the psoas properly while walking and running, but it involves first learning to stand and walk without using the psoas as a structural support. Walking Instructor, Suki Munsell, Ph.D., has developed a re-education program called "Dynamic Walking" whereby one learns to engage the psoas while actively walking.[24] The movement sequence of the psoas as a pendulum is initiated at T12 where the impulse of walking begins and the leg simply follows. Effortless walking starts at the core with a supple, dynamic psoas. With each step, the psoas moves through its full range of motion: neutral, toning, neutral, lengthening. In rhythm with the arms, the legs move asymmetrically, in a cross lateral movement pattern.

SWIMMING: Depending upon the way it is taught and practiced, swimming is an activity that can either create neuro-skeletal problems or release them. Professional swimmers are known to develop shoulder tendonitis and kyphosis. Overriding head and neck righting reflexes by repeatedly tucking the head and/

or rotating the head and arms without moving the trunk eventually results in overdeveloped shoulder muscles that impinge upon the thoracic outlet and distorts the ribcage. These ongoing problems are prevalent in the professional arena. Bob Cooley, director of The Genius of Flexibility Studio, developed "The Swim Stroke" and presented it to the U.S. Olympic Advanced Coaches Seminar in Colorado in 1978. The stroke is based upon natural movement patterns of the arm and shoulder that do not override the head and neck reflexes. The stroke frees the expression and the power of the psoas by allowing the whole core to arc freely with the legs following. By freeing the psoas to release and respond to every breath, swimming becomes a core activity. This stroke includes having the head and eyes slightly out of the water while the spine gently arcs as the psoas lengthens and the legs and feet follow the propulsion of movement similar to a hydrofoil moving across water. The stroke is not imposed upon the body, it develops out of a proprioceptive awareness, which increasingly develops a person's motor skills.

WEIGHT LIFTING & POWER LIFTING: Bodybuilding may be a fashionable activity for sculpting the body; however, the psoas is rarely involved. Bodybuilding is not a process for gaining strength and therefore should not be confused with 'working out' or weightlifting. When a person works out with weights, it is important to have aligned bones and a responsive psoas to be able to transfer weight efficiently and effectively. Otherwise the body will attempt to compensate and multiple problems can arise (such as torn and bruised muscles, tendon and ligament strains, and joint injuries). In contrast, powerlifting focuses on functional strength. To achieve functional strength a person must first increase his or her proprioceptive neuro-pathways. When training having a neutral, supple psoas as well as skeletal proprioception can transform powerlifting into a journey toward maximizing power and strength.

Approaches

YOGA: Various forms of yoga can encourage a limber body and mind. Yet for yoga to be psoas-savvy, correct positioning is essential. How a yoga posture is approached, who is guiding the correction of the posture, and what the ultimate intention is, will determine a positive or negative outcome. Although yoga asanas can potentially stretch specific muscle groups, stimulate organ functioning, improve the breath, and activate the meridian flows (energy pathways through the body), when practiced incorrectly yoga can also overextend joints (the pulling apart of bones at the junctions) as well as stretch and destabilize ligaments. Additionally, the psoas should not be engaged to achieve and maintain a posture. If delicate joints are locked and/or injured, yoga will disrupt proprioception, which will inadvertently impede upon having a healthy psoas. Thus it is crucial for the foundation of every asana to begin with a supple psoas and a centered pelvic basin.

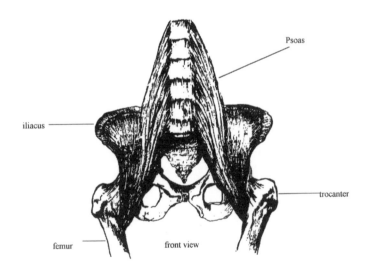

iliacus

Psoas

trocanter

femur   front view

Notes

1. Ida Rolf, *Rolfing: The Integration of the Human Structure* (New York: Harper & Row, 1997), 113.

2. Ibid., 118.

3. Karlfried Graf Von Durkheim, *Hara: The Vital Centre of Man* (London: Unwin Paperbacks, 1977), 17.

4. Mabel Elsworth Todd, *The Thinking Body: A Study of the Balancing Forces of Dynamic Man* (New York: Dance Horizons, Inc., 1978), 62.

5. Michio. Kushi, *The Book of Macrobiotics: The Universal Way of Health and Happiness* (Tokyo: Japan Publications, Inc., 1977), 17.

6. Susan K Campbell, "Inherent Movement Patterns In Man" *Journal of Kinesiology III* (1973), 55.

7. Ibid.

8. Rolf, *Rolfing*, 113.

9. Moshe Feldenkrais, *Body & Mature Behavior: A Study Of Anxiety, Sex, Gravitation & Learning* (New York: International Universities Press, Inc., 1975), 83.

10. Ibid., 87.

11. Ibid., 93.

12. Wilhelm Reich, *The Discovery of the Orgone: The Function of the Orgasm* (New York: Noonday Press, 1961), 275.

13. Therese Bertherat and Carol Bernstein, *The Body Has Its Reasons: Anti-exercise and Self-Awareness* (New York: Avon Books, 1979), 100.

14. Reich, *The Function of the Orgasm*, 110.

15. Feldenkrais, *Body & Mature Behavior*, 156.

16. Ron Kurtz and Hector Prestera, *The Body Reveals: An Illustrated Guide to the Psychology of the Body* (New York: Harper & Row/Quicksilver Books, 1976), 66.

17. Felix Mann, *Acupuncture: The Ancient Chinese Art of Healing and How it Works Scientifically* (New York: Vintage Books, 1973), 47.

Notes

18. Durkheim, *Hara*, 81.

19. Kurts and Prestera, *The Body Reveals*, 72.

20. Campbell, "Inherent Movement Patterns In Man," 59.

21. Feldenkrais, *Body & Mature Behavior*, 150.

22. *Somatics Magazine/Journal*, "A Somatics Interview with Judith Aston."

23. Bob Cooley, "East-West Dance Forms" (1976).

24. Suki Munsell, *Dynamic Health & Fitness: Mastering Your Vitality, http://
    ~www.dynamicvitality.com.*

Bibliography

Alexander, F. Matthias. *The Use of the Self*. California: Centerline Press, 1984.

Bertherat, Therese and Carol Bernstein. *The Body Has Its Reasons: Anti-exercise and Self-Awareness*. New York: Avon Books, 1979.

Campbell, Susan K. "Inherent Movement Patterns In Man," *Journal of Kinesiology III, 1973.*

Cooley, Bob. "East-West Dance Forms" Boston: The Moving Center, Inc., 1976.

Durkheim, Karlfried Graf Von. *Hara: The Vital Centre of Man.* Mandala ed. London: Unwin Paperbacks, 1977.

Feitis, Rosemary. *Ida Rolf Talks About Rolfing & Physical Reality*. New York: Harper & Row, 1978.

Feldenkrais, Moshe. *Body & Mature Behavior: A Study Of Anxiety, Sex, Gravitation & Learning.* 3rd ed. New York: International Universities Press, Inc., 1975.

Gershon, Michael D., M.D. *The Second Brain.* New York: HarperCollins, Inc.,1998.

Kent, Christine Ann. *Saving the Whole Woman: Natural Alternatives to Surgery for Pelvic Organ Prolapse and Urinary Incontinence.* 2nd ed. Albuquerque: Bridgeworks, Inc., 2008.

Kurtz, Ron and Hector Prestera, M.D. *The Body Reveals: An Illustrated Guide to the Psychology of the Body*. New York: Harper & Row/Quicksilver Books, 1976.

Kushi, Michio. *The Book of Macrobiotics: The Universal Way of Health and Happiness*. Tokyo: Japan Publications, Inc., 1977.

Mann, Felix, M.B. *Acupuncture: The Ancient Chinese Art of Healing and How it Works Scientifically*. New York: Vintage Books, 1973.

Reich, Wilhelm, M.D. *The Discovery of the Orgone: The Function of the Orgasm.* 3rd ed. New York: Noonday Press, 1961.

Rolf, Ida P, Ph.D. *Rolfing: The Integration of the Human Structure*. New York: Harper & Row, 1977.

Somatics Magazine/Journal, "A Somatics Interview with Judith Aston," autumn 1980.

Sweigard, Lulu. *Human Movement Potential: Its Ideokinetic Facilitation*. New York: Harper & Row, 1974.

Todd, Mabel Elsworth. *The Thinking Body: A Study of the Balancing Forces of Dynamic Man*. New York: Dance Horizons, Inc., 1978.

About The Author

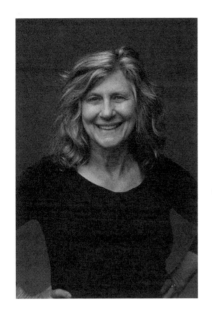

Liz Koch is an international teacher and author with over 30 years experience working with and specializing in the iliopsoas muscle. Recognized by colleagues in the movement, wellness, and fitness professions as an authority on the core muscle of the human body, Liz Koch is an educator, working with both laypersons and professionals.

Liz Koch is the author of *The Psoas Book; Core Awareness: Enhancing Yoga*, Pilates, Exercise & Dance (1st edition by Guinea Pig Publications 2003, 2nd edition by North Atlantic Books, released Fall 2012); *Unraveling Scoliosis CD; Psoas & Back Pain CD;* and a contributing author of *Maiden, Mother, Crone: Our Pleasure Playlist.*

Liz Koch is the creator of *Core Awareness,*™ which is a somatic approach to deepening the experience of the human core. Beginning with the core muscle, the iliopsoas, *Core Awareness*™ focuses attention on sensation as a means for maturing and developing the proprioceptive nervous system, which is responsible for skeletal alignment, balance and orientation. For books, articles, podcasts, tele-classes, and workshop information visit www.coreawareness.com.

Liz Koch's writing is featured in *Yoga Journal*, *Positive Health*, *Massage & Bodywork, Vegetarian Time, Yoga & Health, Midwifery Today*, and *Massage Magazine* as well as numerous small health and wellness publications. Serving her community by developing a health and wellness program for Way Of Life, Liz Koch writes a monthly newsletter available online (www.wayoflife.net).

Liz Koch is recognized by the National Certification Board for Therapeutic Massage & Bodywork (NCBTMB) as an approved continuing education provider. She is also a member of the International Movement Educators Association (IMEA).